Living with Methylisothiazolinone Allergy
The Complete Guide

by

Alex Gazzola

Text copyright © 2018 Alex Gazzola

All rights reserved and asserted in accordance with the Copyright, Designs and Patents Act 1988

No part of this book may be transmitted, shared or reproduced in any form or by any means, including via print, electronic or broadcast media, without the written permission of the author.

The author has made every effort to ensure the accuracy of the content, but cannot guarantee it is free of inadvertent errors, nor that it will remain current.

The author makes no warranty of any kind with regard to the content as it stands, and disclaims all liabilities for it, including but not limited to any loss occasioned to any person acting or refraining from action as a result of the content.

The book is *not* intended as a substitute for professional medical advice, and doctors should always be consulted.

No responsibility can be taken for the content of third-party websites or resources referred to or recommended in the text.

First printing January 2019

ISBN: 9781790916757

Contents

About the author	*v*
Author's note	*vii*
Introduction: a history of MI	*ix*
1. What is MI?	1
2. Allergy testing and diagnosis	7
3. Cosmetic sense: safe toiletries	17
4. Home sense: safe household products	29
5. Avoiding exposure	39
6. Skin health, skin reactions	55
7. Other allergies	67
8. Emotional health	75
Conclusion: the outlook	*91*
Resources	*95*
Glossary	*99*
Acknowledgements	*105*
Index	*107*

About the author

Alex Gazzola has been a health writer for over twenty years, and now specializes in gut health, allergies and other food and environmental sensitivities. He is the author of five print books — including *Living With Food Intolerance*, and *IBS: Dietary Advice to Calm Your Gut* — and three e-books for aspiring writers. He has contributed to magazines and newspapers in over twenty countries, as well as specialist allergy publications both in print and online. He edits the Methylisothiazolinone Free (www.mi-free.com) and Allergy Insight (www.allergy-insight.com) websites.

Author's note

This book is aimed at an international readership of people dealing with the everyday and long-term consequences of living with allergy to methylisothiazolinone (MI) and related isothiazolinone preservatives — whether that allergy is suspected or confirmed, whether the reader is a patient, parent or carer.

Your personal circumstances and degree of interest in the subject will determine which chapters may or may not be relevant or of value to you.

The Introduction which follows provides background to the use of isothiazolinones, giving recent historical context to what has become a modern-day health epidemic. There's no escaping the fact that the biography of these preservatives is a complex one, and while I've simplified it for the purposes of this short book, you may wish to skip the section entirely as it is not essential to understanding what comes later.

Similarly, chapter 2 — which deals with tests and diagnoses — is arguably optional to those who already have a medical confirmation from a dermatologist that they or their child has an MI allergy, although you may still find it useful.

Many coming to this book will be looking for safe product recommendations, and while there are a number of suggestions throughout, readers are urged to double-check more up-to-date lists provided on the Methylisothiazolinone Free website (www.mi-free.com) and other resources mentioned. Even then, remember that mistakes can be made, formulations and company policies change regularly, and 100% guarantees are impossible.

As is the case with any health book, this one cannot diagnose any medical condition. Its intention is to support and inform, but it cannot replace the expertise that only a qualified doctor, allergist or dermatologist can provide.

Note that the expression 'MI free' is sometimes used, and should generally be taken to mean isothiazolinone-free unless specified.

Note too that the book is written by a user of British English, in the knowledge that the bulk of its readers will be users of American English. I've tended towards using the latter's spelling preferences, and trust the resulting 'Brimerican' English won't compromise legibility or clarity for either group of readers, or indeed others. Please forgive any inconsistencies.

Feedback on the book — and specifically on what can be improved in future editions — would be most welcome. You can contact me at info@mi-free.com.

Alex Gazzola

Introduction: a history of MI

Allergy to the group of preservatives known as isothiazolinones first emerged as an occupational disease in the early eighties. The most well-known isothiazolinone preservative nowadays is methylisothiazolinone (MI), but those first reports involved lesser-known relatives of methylisothiazolinone — for instance, benzisothiazolinone (BIT) allergy in a laborer in a rubber factory, and octylisothiazolinone (OIT) allergy among shoe factory workers.

Three further case reports were published in the journal *Contact Dermatitis* in February 1985. Very unluckily, one of the three individuals was said to have been sensitized to isothiazolinones via a patch test. The allergies of the other two were caused by exposure to a moisturizing cream containing both MI and another isothiazolinone, called methylchloroisothiazolinone (MCI). A mix of MI / MCI in a ratio of roughly 1:3, known by the trade name Kathon CG, had been used in European cosmetics since the mid-seventies, and in the US since the early eighties, and these cases appear to have been the first non-occupational ones reported.

In the late eighties, the problem escalated. More papers appeared in specialist journals, a number of them authored or co-authored by the Dutch dermatologist Anton C de Groot.

In 1987, de Groot published results revealing that 3.3% of those patch-tested for suspected contact dermatitis had Kathon CG allergy.

"Contact allergy to Kathon CG is common," he wrote of this new epidemic. "Sensitisation usually occurs from creams and lotions applied to damaged skin, but some become sensitised by cosmetic products used on healthy skin, especially on the face and around the eyes."

The following year he dubbed Kathon CG "by far the most important cosmetic allergen", and the year after that, in a paper published in the medical journal *The Lancet*, titled *Isothiazolinone preservative: cause of a continuing epidemic of cosmetic dermatitis*, he offered the view that "Most cases [of contact allergy] have been caused by products of the 'leave-on' variety, such as moisturising creams. The use of isothiazolinone preservative in such products should be abandoned."

It was in 1989 that this warning was issued.

Thirty years on, it has yet to be fully acted upon worldwide.

The nineties

Instead of being "abandoned", the use of the MI / MCI blend was more tightly regulated, with stricter limits on the quantities cosmetic formulators could use. The expert view was that lax controls over permitted concentrations had caused the epidemic.

In 1992, a panel from the Cosmetic Ingredient Review (CIR) — a US-based professional body assessing cosmetic ingredient safety — concluded that the MI / MCI blend could be safely used in rinse-off products at a concentration not exceeding 15ppm (15 parts per million — or 0.0015%) and in leave-on products at 7.5ppm.

This reduction, from the previous limit of 30ppm, took some sting out of the epidemic, but did not halt it by any means.

At around this time, another preservative, called methyldibromo glutaronitrile (MDBGN), had become increasingly popular. This had been introduced in the mid-eighties and was touted as a less sensitizing alternative to MI / MCI.

It turned out to be anything but.

Allergy to MDBGN sky-rocketed through the nineties. A study by the European Environmental & Contact Dermatitis Research Group, published in the journal *Contact Dermatitis* in 2002, showed that the prevalence of allergy to it rose from 0.7% in 1991 to 3.5% in 2000.

This prompted a drawn-out safety review, the end result of which was a decision to withdraw MDBGN, but it still took some years for the preservative to be outlawed in Europe, first in leave-on cosmetics in 2005, then in rinse-off by 2007. (It remains permitted in the US and elsewhere, though appears to be infrequently used.)

The new millennium

Preservatives were suddenly under intense scrutiny.

The class of preservatives known as parabens also came under suspicion, after research was published revealing traces of them had been found in women's breast tissue, and linking the preservatives' use in underarm deodorants and anti-perspirants to breast cancer.

But other studies found no association, and there continues to be disagreement on the matter to this day, despite there being no unequivocal and convincing evidence linking the two.

What has also endured has been the damage to parabens' reputation — it took hold then, it remains now, and it was a key reason behind the increasing use of MI / MCI, at the time perceived by some to be a safer alternative.

In 2000, MI as a 'standalone' preservative was authorized for use in industrial products, without any maximum limiting threshold.

Despite the emergence of several occupational cases of MI allergy which followed this decision, it was still widely believed that, of the two main isothiazolinone preservatives, MCI was the evil 'Hyde' to the more benevolent 'Jekyll' of MI.

In other words, it was thought that MCI was the more dangerous sensitizer, with an extreme allergenic potency, highly capable of triggering allergy and loss of tolerance — in some cases even after just a single exposure.

This, in part, led to a decision being taken in Europe in 2005 to permit the use of MI as a cosmetic preservative in its own right; previously, it had only been used in combination with MCI in the Kathon CG blend.

But there was a catch ...

The MI problem

As a weaker preservative, MI had to be used in higher concentrations in order to be effective; consequently, 100ppm were permitted across all cosmetics — roughly 25 and 50 times greater than the concentration allowed when used in combination with MCI in Kathon CG, in rinse-off and leave-on cosmetics respectively.

North America followed suit. In 2008, a panel from the CIR released an assessment concluding that MI was safe to use at the same concentration. This was published in the *International Journal of Toxicology* in 2010, and as the abstract read: "Although recognising that MIT [another abbreviation for MI] was a sensitizer in both animal and human studies, the panel concluded that there is a threshold dose response and that cosmetic products formulated to contain concentrations … at 100ppm (0.01%) or less would not be expected to pose a sensitization risk."

But by the same year, alarm bells were ringing loudly elsewhere. There were reports of young children being sensitized to MI through its use in moist tissues or 'wet wipes' — as well as an increase in sensitizations through everyday cosmetics, particularly in young to middle-aged women.

Among those concerned about moist toilet tissue was dermatologist Dr Juan García-Gavin. Writing in *Archives of Dermatology* in 2010, he warned that this 'new' standalone MI preservative may not be the solution to the isothiazolinone allergy problem at all.

In the next couple of years, the picture became clearer and experts began to gather in agreement around a wretched conclusion: the increase in frequency of use of MI was leading to more and more allergy.

To the present day …

In early 2013, MI earned the dubious honor of being named 'Allergen of the Year', as awarded by the American Contact Dermatitis Society.

Just weeks before that announcement, Margarida Gonçalo, president of the European Society of Contact Dermatitis, formally wrote to the European Commission (EC) to request investigations into the preservative's safety. "This new epidemic of allergic contact dermatitis from isothiazolinones is causing harm to European citizens," she wrote. "Urgent action is required."

In an article Gonçalo later submitted to the journal *Contact Dermatitis*, she outlined that the matter had been repeatedly raised internally with the EC's Directorate-General for Health and Food Safety "for over a year" beforehand, but was "not considered a priority by the risk managers", adding that "the slow process of risk assessment, risk management and intervention will result in continuing harm".

The EC came under further fire. Here was Dr Ian White, consultant dermatologist at St John's Institute of Dermatology in the UK: "Bluntly, I think the European Commission has been negligent over this. They have had warning after warning. If it was food there would have been action."

The Scientific Committee on Consumer Safety, the EC's independent expert committee, announced support for the prohibition of methylisothiazolinone in leave-on cosmetics, and a reduction of its permitted concentration in rinse-off products from 100ppm to 15ppm.

Cosmetics Europe (CE), the European personal care umbrella association for cosmetic manufacturers, urged its members not to wait for regulation to be passed — but instead, to remove MI from its leave-on cosmetics as soon as possible.

CE was wise to make this recommendation, as regulation was not introduced quickly. Although it is necessary to give cosmetics manufacturers time to reformulate their products, the MI / MCI blend was effectively banned from leave-on cosmetics only in April 2016, and MI in February 2017 — but solely in the EU, not elsewhere. In rinse-off products, a reduced maximum concentration of 15ppm for MI came into effect in 2018.

There are those who understandably feel that slow decision-making by those charged with managing public health, teamed with their failure to fully assess the sensitizing potential of the isothiazolinone preservatives, have led to around 1.5% of the population becoming allergic to one or more of these common ingredients.

That, very sadly and needlessly, is where we are.

And where we are is a place where millions of people have isothiazolinone allergy — many of them undiagnosed — with most of them needing help.

1. What is MI?

MI is **methylisothiazolinone** — an effective synthetic preservative, used in consumer products such as toiletries, cosmetics and baby wipes to prevent the growth of bacteria and molds, thereby extending products' shelf life and usage, and protecting consumers against exposure to harmful organisms.

A related preservative — **methylchloroisothiazolinone**, or **MCI** — is also used in cosmetics, but usually only in a blend with MI, sometimes called Kathon CG (CG stands for 'cosmetic grade'), which is a mixture of three parts MCI to one part MI.

MCI *cannot* be used in cosmetics independently of MI, at least in Europe.

MI and MCI are typically used in water-based or water-containing products, such as lotions or gels. (Water normally goes by the name 'aqua' in lists of ingredients, and is often named first.)

MI was named Allergen of the Year in 2013.

Both MI and MCI may also be found in many household products, such as fabric conditioners and dishwashing liquids, where they are sometimes (but not always) labeled or declared. Such products may also contain other types of so-called isothiazolinones, such as **benzisothiazolinone (BIT)** and **octylisothiazolinone (OIT)**, which are increasingly common members of the same 'family'.

Household paints are very likely to contain several isothiazolinones, but paints are generally not required to be labeled with ingredients unless present above a certain threshold level.

All these preservatives are widely used in various industries too — such as engineering, textiles, paper and aviation.

Increasing use of MI

Although there are now signs of a downturn, the use of MI has generally increased in cosmetics during the last ten or 15 years.

There appear to be several reasons for this:

1. Concern over a class of preservatives called parabens, the use of which some have suggested could increase the risk of breast cancer, although this has *not* been scientifically proved. In response to this public misperception, many manufacturers have sought to use alternative preservatives — among them MI.

2. Earlier concern about the safety of MCI resulted in a reduction in the use of the MI / MCI blend, meaning that some manufacturers chose to use MI only, once it had been authorized, and sometimes in very high concentrations, given that MI is the weaker preservative of the two and is required in greater quantity in order to kill bacteria and molds.

3. Effectiveness — the isothiazolinone preservatives happen to be very good at their job, and they work across a wide range of pH values too.

Allergy to MI

Allergies to many kinds of sensitizers have been on the increase worldwide for some years, and in line with this rise in reactions to foods, pollens, dust mites, fragrances and other materials, allergy to methylisothiazolinone and its relatives has also gone up.

An allergy is essentially a hypersensitivity reaction caused by the immune system — the system of cells, tissues and organs in the body responsible for protecting it from outside 'invaders', and preventing infection from bacteria or parasites.

In an allergic reaction, the immune system mistakenly regards an external environmental trigger as a dangerous threat, and reacts defensively.

A food allergy, for example, is what immunologists call a type I reaction, in which the response is fast, involving the release of histamine and other chemicals in the body in an attempt to defend against the perceived intruder. It results in unpleasant and sometimes serious symptoms such as nettle rash, swollen lips and tongue, and wheezing.

A skin allergy to a cosmetic ingredient is usually a type IV reaction, in this case called allergic contact dermatitis (ACD).

Here, the sensitizing agent — in this case, the isothiazolinone preservative — reacts with a protein in the skin to produce a 'conjugate' which the immune system marks out as 'foreign'.

Once this sensitization has taken place, subsequent exposures will trigger a reaction.

The full biochemical response is complex, but inflammatory in nature, eventually leading to the typical symptoms associated with ACD.

Allergy to MI and/or other isothiazolinones effects up to 1.5% of the population, the considerable majority female.

Women seem disproportionately affected, almost certainly because they use more cosmetics, and are exposed to more cosmetic and other household chemicals due to generally performing more childcare and cleaning duties than male counterparts.

Male skin is also a little thicker than female skin, and this could well play a role in the statistical imbalance, as might the thinning of women's skin during menopause.

Symptoms of MI allergy

There are many potential symptoms, and those with allergy to MI and related isothiazolinones will experience one or more of them, but not necessarily all.

It will vary depending on the type of exposure and the individual. No two people's experiences are ever exactly alike, and the degree of severity will also differ.

Time of onset following exposure can also vary: from a number of hours to a few days.

Symptoms can persist for many weeks. They include:

- redness / rashes;
- inflammation;
- itchiness / irritation;
- stinging;
- swelling (eg of eyelids);
- blistering / pustules;
- scaly and flaky skin.

These symptoms of eczema and dermatitis can appear anywhere on the body, but sites typically affected include the fingers and hands, around the eyes and mouth, and in babies, the diaper area. These tend to be the areas where most cosmetics are handled, used or applied — as well as parts of the body regularly touched by the hands.

Because the isothiazolinones are volatile, they can become airborne — for instance, from paint applied to walls, as it dries and off-gases or vaporises, but also from surface tops wiped with detergent — and subsequent inhalation and exposure can also trigger unpleasant symptoms, especially in those with other allergic diseases such as asthma.

When this happens — that is, when exposure and reaction is through a non-skin route — it is called systemic contact dermatitis.

As well as symptoms of the skin, others reported include nausea, headaches, stinging in the eyes, muscular spasms and neurological (nerve) pain.

There have been a few anecdotally reported cases of anaphylaxis, the most severe of all allergic reactions, which require adrenaline / epinephrine and hospital treatment — but these are very rare.

It's important to recognize that all these symptoms can also be symptoms of other allergies, and in some cases of other conditions.

Do not necessarily assume that, just because you are experiencing them or have experienced some of them in the past, that you are definitely allergic to isothiazolinones.

To be sure, you must undergo skin patch testing ...

2. Allergy testing and diagnosis

Before addressing what you *should* do in order to seek a proper diagnosis of MI allergy — or indeed any other allergy — it's important to emphasize what you *shouldn't* do.

Self diagnosis

Who, in this great internet age, can honestly hold up their hand and swear that they have never used 'Dr Google' to search the world wide web for symptoms and their possible causes?

It's understandable. With millions of pages of information at our fingertips, the temptation can be too much to resist. But even if what you uncover is reliable and accurate — and in the unedited 'wild west' of the web, there is an unacceptable risk that it is not — it still cannot and will not give you a definitive answer to what might be troubling you or your child's skin and health.

Never self-diagnose any allergy, including to MI or MCI. It is unreliable.

It is human nature to look for evidence in support of something we have come to suspect or believe. For instance, once we form and have settled on a certain political view, we pay more attention to those supporting or promoting that view, than we do to those who might challenge it.

Once we begin to indulge in a superstition — such as wearing a lucky T-shirt for certain occasions, such as a sporting event — we persist with it for years, seeking reassurance from times when it 'works', and finding excuses for times when it doesn't.

It is satisfying and legitimizing to prove ourselves right; it is destabilizing and upsetting to prove ourselves wrong. Our inclination is to aim for the former. But it's a very risky practice, not least when it comes to our health.

Scientists and medics do not work like this. They can't. If a scientific result questions their understanding of a medical issue or matter, they may seek to replicate it — but once they've succeeded they do everything in their power to challenge it. This is because the truth can withstand any test at all.

Any suspicion you have must always be properly investigated and challenged. And for that, you need help.

Your doctor

A doctor will certainly listen to your suspicions, if you have them, and your symptoms, of course, but will also consider your wider clinical history and look for alternative possibilities. He or she will examine your skin.

A doctor will also ask you questions, so it pays to be prepared for these in advance, as consultations can be quick and it's easy to forget patterns of symptoms and experiences.

If it helps in the run-up to your appointment, keep a 'reaction diary' of exposure and symptoms — making a note of what you use or expose your skin to, be it cosmetics, household products, beauty treatments, a public swimming pool, materials at work, and so on, and what the response of your skin is. What you write may not reveal much to you, and no apparent pattern may emerge, but specialists can sometimes see things which you can't. Record every detail as accurately as possible and take pictures on your phone.

Some questions you may be asked include:

- Do the symptoms come and go, or are they persistent or long-term?
- Do they appear on certain parts of the body, or anywhere and everywhere?
- Have you taken anything for them, or applied anything new to your skin?
- Has anything in your day-to-day routine changed in recent weeks?
- Have you undergone any major life upheaval in recent weeks or months?

It may be an allergy; it may not. If your doctor thinks it could be, he or she may refer you for patch testing.

Patch testing

This is a specialist medical procedure used to investigate whether any skin-based symptoms you are experiencing might be aggravated or caused by an allergy to a substance to which it is being exposed.

The exposure can come through cosmetics, toiletries, household detergents and other domestic products, as well as clothing, pollen, pollutants, or other materials in your daily environment, such as leather, metal, rubber, plastics and so on.

Patch testing is conducted by dermatologists, allergists and dermatological nurses, and its aim is to discover the exact causes of your symptoms — whether or not they are due to allergy, and if so, what the triggers might be.

Anyone can undergo patch testing, but there are some contra-indications — that is, if you are pregnant or breastfeeding, have severe eczema on your back, are taking immuno-suppressant medication, or taking certain steroids.

Materials and information

So that they can also be tested, if considered appropriate, you may be asked to bring along samples of items with which you are in regular contact — such as particular cosmetics (including nail varnish, scents, moisturizers, sun creams), household products (fabric softeners, detergents), and materials you are exposed to at work.

This is particularly important for people such as decorators, hairdressers, beauticians, factory workers and indeed medical workers themselves.

The ingredients of some of these materials may not always be disclosed or easily available to you. Try to ascertain them beforehand, if you can. Many products feature customer helpline numbers on their labels.

Material Safety Data Sheets

Each industrial, detergent or non-cosmetic material should have a material safety data sheet (MSDS) associated with it.

An MSDS — also called a product safety data sheet or, simply, safety data sheet (SDS) — is a document outlining hazard information.

You can sometimes track down a MSDS online at the manufacturer's website, and it may (or may not) disclose full or partial ingredients. Such documents, however, are not intended for general consumers, but rather for relevant occupational workers, risk assessors and health and safety analysts. They may not be particularly reader friendly, in other words.

It's also worth making direct enquiries with manufacturers or health and safety officers at your place of work, as they are likely to have experience in sourcing full ingredients of any products used on the premises, such as detergents, adhesives, printer inks, coolants, fertilizers and many more.

What is involved?

The patch testing process itself involves applying small amounts of substances to your skin, usually along the top of your back, in the form of small discs or patches infused with the test substances, and which are fixed in place with medical tape.

You will be asked to not expose your back to the sun or a sunlamp for several weeks before your first appointment.

Men with hairy backs may be wise to carefully shave the day before their appointment, which can also mean eventual patch removal is less painful. Waxing should be avoided.

You will be advised to wear old clothing as the process can stain.

With patches on your back, front-buttoning tops (eg shirts, blouses) will be easier to put back on than over-the-head ones (eg sweaters).

Bring along any medication you are taking, even over-the-counter medicines, as well as prescription drugs, and any supplements (liquid or tablet) which you take regularly.

Anything from around twenty to over a hundred substances may be tested, depending on your particular circumstances and the chemicals you may regularly be exposed to. Usually, a set 'baseline' series will be applied to all patients, plus others which are specific and appropriate to you, as an individual.

The patches themselves will be aligned in one or more grids and marked carefully with inks on your back in order to identify each potential allergen.

You should wear these for two days, or as long as directed, ensuring you keep your back completely dry. Swimming or showering is not permitted. Keep yourself clean elsewhere with a washcloth, and take extreme care if taking a shallow bath.

Exercise and sun exposure are best avoided too — sweating can loosen the adhesives.

After two days, you will be asked to attend a second appointment, and the patches will be removed and sites examined.

Another two days later, you will be asked to attend a third appointment and your dermatologist will further examine all the patch sites for potential allergies.

Results

Results can only be interpreted reliably by experienced dermatologists.

Many reactions will be negative. Do not be despondent if *all* tests are negative. This is still a useful result, which will bring your doctors a step closer to identifying what the actual causes or culprits are.

Some may be uncertain.

Some may be due to irritation, rather than allergy — in other words, your skin may respond to a substance simply because it doesn't 'like' being exposed to it for four days, but not because it is allergic, or would react to it under normal circumstances, or with a fleeting exposure. Essentially, an irritant reaction is one which is prominently symptomatic after 48 hours, but resolves noticeably after 96 hours.

But one or more may be positive — be it weakly, strongly, or extremely positive. Positive allergic reactions show up as elevated pink or red patches, and the stronger ones may be blistered. An allergic reaction is likely to be more severe after 96 hours than it is at 48 hours, as it is slower to develop. Your dermatologist will probably make a firm diagnosis of allergic contact dermatitis, or allergic contact eczema — be it to MI / MCI and/or to other chemicals or substances.

Side effects

Obviously, positive and perhaps irritant reactions will come with the side effects of itching and reddening at the application sites. Skin under patches may blister if strongly positive.

Some reactions may last up to a month, but will then fade, and if you have had recurrent flare-ups of eczema during your life, then you may find that these could be aggravated during and after the patch testing. Again, this should fade.

More serious side effects — change in pigment, or infection, or scarring — are extremely rare.

Top tips …

- If seeing a private dermatologist, ensure he or she is a member of an established, well-regarded professional association — such as the American Contact Dermatitis Society (ACDS). For other associations, see Resources (page 95). (Member dermatologists can often access helpful databases of up-to-date 'safe' product lists.)

- If you suspect MI / MCI allergy, ensure that the patch test you are undertaking is extensive, and contains patches for both MI in isolation, and MI / MCI combined. It is important to test MI on its own as there may be insufficient in the MI / MCI combination to elicit a reaction, and not all who are allergic to MI react to MCI too. Check with the professional conducting the test that this is the case. One panel test, the T.R.U.E. Test, contains only the MI / MCI mix by default, and not MI. But the ACDS-recommended core allergen series panels *do* include MI among their 80 allergens (NAC-80 — The North American 80 Comprehensive Series).

- There are panels for certain jobs or industries (eg 'hairdressing'), so ensure that such a panel is included if appropriate to you.

- Ask a partner for help getting dressed if you're concerned about dislodging the patches on your back. Button-up shirts and cardigans might be safer and easier to get on than T-shirts or sweaters that have to go over your head.

- Ask your dermatologist or pharmacist for some hypoallergenic microporous adhesive tape in case any of the patches loosen. In the UK, Micropore or Scanpor are two options.

- Do not leave the clinic or surgery without a complete list of all the ingredients tested and the results — especially of any positives, if they include others in addition to MI / MCI. You will need to refer to these in the weeks, months and indeed years to come.

- Rarely, reactions can be unusually delayed and may occur after your dermatologist has seen you to examine your results — even, exceptionally, after up to two weeks. Do let your practitioner know if this happens, and perhaps ask a partner or friend to take a photograph of your back, including a close-up of the reaction itself, in case there is a further delay between the reaction and the next available appointment slot when you can be seen.

Diagnosis

If you receive a diagnosis of MI / MCI allergy (and perhaps additional allergies to other ingredients) most of the advice you will be given will focus on avoidance.

You will probably be given a leaflet or short guide, which will contain basic information, but is unlikely to cover all aspects you need to consider in the longer-term.

Some doctors will give you lists of products, but always check in case of recent ingredient changes.

Your dermatologist may also prescribe some short-term medications if your ACD is severe: these may include steroids and immuno-suppressants to treat existing symptoms and any additional ones which developed as a result of patch testing. Always double-check that any topical treatments are free of your newly-discovered allergens! We will return to medications in chapter 6.

You should also receive some advice on looking after your skin: good skin care will focus on regularly using safe emollients (moisturizers) and skin protection. In the UK and EU, all leave-on emollients are MI- and MCI-free, but this is not yet the case in North America, Australia and New Zealand, for example. It may not be necessary to completely overhaul your skincare or beauty routine, but some products may well have to go.

The good news is that you are now armed with information to address the causes of the problems, and relieve the symptoms.

Misdiagnoses

Many diagnosed with MI allergy relate that they were previously misdiagnosed with any number of skin diseases and conditions, such as rosacea, psoriasis, blepharitis, scabies, impetigo or others.

Others are told they may have autoimmune conditions (such as Sjögren's syndrome, rheumatoid arthritis, lupus) or that their skincare maintenance or personal hygiene is poor.

All this can be frustrating, stressful and upsetting.

If you are not satisfied with the investigations and diagnosis you receive, you must ask for a second opinion from an alternative specialist. Ask for patch testing to be conducted if it has been denied to you and you have good reasons to suspect contact allergies.

3. Cosmetic sense: safe toiletries

What *is* a cosmetic?

When it comes to allergy to cosmetic ingredients, it's important to be clear and specific.

So: a cosmetic is a preparation which is applied to parts of the body in order to clean, fragrance, deodorize, condition or protect them, or change their appearance.

These parts of the body include the obvious areas — such as the skin and hair — but also the lips, nails, oral cavity, external genital organs and anal region.

While many of us consider cosmetics to essentially mean make-up, they do in fact incorporate creams, lotions, soaps, cleansers, gels, perfumes, toothpastes, mouthwashes, sunscreen, vaginal washes, lubricants, moistened toilet paper and much more besides.

Ingredients labels

Lists of ingredients on cosmetics can be intimidating to anyone not familiar with chemistry, and it's not surprising many people do not even attempt to read them.

However, if you have been diagnosed with an allergy to an ingredient used in cosmetics, it is essential you make the effort to decipher the label.

Preservatives such as methylisothiazolinone and methylchloroisothiazolinone are used in very small quantities relative to other ingredients. Because ingredients are generally declared in descending order of quantity, you will typically find them towards the end of an ingredients list.

You should see those very words — methylchloroisothiazolinone, methylchloroisothiazolinone — in full, and *not* the abbreviations MI or MCI.

Where abbreviations *are* sometimes used is in a 'free from' claim — ie "MI Free" or "free from MI / MCI" — made elsewhere on the packaging. These claims are increasingly being adopted by natural brands, but are disliked by many in the mainstream cosmetic industry, and regulation against their use is tightening in the EU. Even if you see such a claim, double check the ingredients list to be sure, or for other allergens or ingredients you need to avoid.

Note that some ingredient names which may resemble an isothiazolinone preservative — such as methylparaben, isomethylionone, methylpropanediol — should be safe, assuming you don't have an allergy to them specifically. See the Glossary (page 99) for other examples.

Outside the EU, you may still sometimes see the expression Kathon CG on cosmetics — the brand name for the MI / MCI blend. Other terms / trade names — again given in the Glossary — are rare, at least on cosmetics.

No isothiazolinone preservative other than MI or MCI is permitted for cosmetic use in the EU or in Australia and New Zealand, though you can never drop your guard. At least one such case has been reported: recently, benzisothiazolinone (BIT) was used illegally in a skin cleanser by Australian brand Skin Physics, and it may have contributed to an extreme reaction in a consumer in New Zealand in late 2017.

In the US, the brand Puracy uses BIT in some of its hand soaps, which is extremely unusual.

Cosmetics in America are regulated by the Food & Drug Administration (FDA), but the rules are widely considered extremely lightweight among cosmetic scientists and international regulators — certainly so relative to the far stricter regulations in place in the UK and EU.

For instance, in Europe, products have to undergo microbial challenge tests, be properly registered before being placed on the market, have serious reactions to them notified to appropriate authorities, and more.

In the US, you can literally make a potion today, and sell it tomorrow.

The EU is stringent about what can and can't go into cosmetics: it bans around ten thousand ingredients.

The US, however, bans only a few dozen.

That said, ingredients must be listed in the US, although there are two exceptions specified by the FDA which are worth bearing in mind:

1. Soap bars which only clean, and have no other claimed or intended purpose (such as moisturization), do *not* need to be labeled. It is rare to find MI / MCI in a bar of soap — but *not* unheard of. Do not risk using anything unlabeled, particularly if you have other allergies.

2. So called incidental ingredients need not be declared. These include the ingredients of a particular ingredient present at an 'insignificant level' in the finished product. Theoretically, this could include MI / MCI. See Parfum / fragrance, overleaf.

You may find that some products — lip sticks, lip balms — are too small to carry legible ingredients labeling, in which case enquire at the point of sale, as ingredients should be made available to you via a leaflet or an online source in such a case.

If you see a cosmetic with the preservative ingredient given simply as 'preservative', you should avoid. It could be an isothiazolinone, or a blend which contains one.

Parfum / fragrance

Many cosmetics are scented in some way.

Even those which are labeled 'fragrance free' may contain ingredients added to 'mask' the scent of other ingredients, some of which may otherwise be unpleasant to the human nose.

Some brands choose to individually list the fragrance components present in their products, and this may include both essential oils and the full chemical names of the sometimes synthetic aromatic compounds used.

Others may use the expressions 'parfum' or 'fragrance' and not give much more information than that.

In the US, there is a trade secret exemption, whereby manufacturers can legally withhold further details on the fragrance blend used.

In the EU, some additional information on certain fragrance components must be provided, although manufacturers are still permitted to avoid fully disclosing what may be in their 'parfum'.

All this presents two potential stumbling blocks to those allergic to MI / MCI.

MI / MCI in fragrance

There has been a lot of concern throughout the online MI-allergy community about the possibility that fragrance ingredients — sold to manufacturers by specialist suppliers — might themselves be preserved with isothiazolinones.

The source of this worry has been a list made available by The International Fragrance Association (IFRA) (www.ifraorg.org/en/ingredients), which has voluntarily disclosed a complete register of materials used in fragrance compounds worldwide. They total around 4,000 — and include MI, MCI, the MI / MCI blend and indeed BIT.

So the question is: can an isothiazolinone be 'hiding' in the expression 'parfum' or 'fragrance' on an ingredient label?

The answer would seem to be yes, but there are considerations to keep in mind.

First, essential oils need no preservation, so we could arguably assume that any 'pure' essential oils should not contain preservatives of any kind. If essential oils are all a manufacturer uses in its formulations for fragrancing, then the risk appears minuscule.

Second, even if a fragrance ingredient *is* preserved with an isothiazolinone preservative, because it (the fragrance) is used in such small amounts in most everyday cosmetics, any trace content would be further diluted to such a degree as to be almost negligible, and unlikely to trigger a reaction.

The exception? The greatest risk would appear to be fragrances, perfumes or eaux de toilettes themselves, which are sprayed onto the skin.

You may also wish to 'play safe' with leave-on cosmetics containing unidentified parfum or fragrance, especially any used around delicate areas, such as the eyes.

With rinse-off cosmetics — such as shower gels — it is thought extremely unlikely you will react to minute traces of isothiazolinone 'hiding' in a fragrance compound.

All that said, sensitivities can vary hugely, and different individuals' reactions are dependent on their own particular tolerance thresholds.

Furthermore, many people will be additionally allergic to some fragrance components, in their own right, having perhaps been diagnosed with both sets of allergies at the same time through their patch tests. We will return to this in chapter 7.

Hypoallergenic cosmetics

What does 'hypoallergenic' actually mean?

It means that a manufacturer which uses the term for one of its products believes — or at least *should* believe — that the product is less likely to trigger allergies in consumers than other, 'non hypoallergenic' products.

There is a lot of skepticism about the term: it "means whatever a particular company wants it to mean", is the US FDA's own view. It is *not* legally defined, then, and so is not regulated in any way.

Furthermore, 'hypoallergenic' cannot mean 'non allergenic' — there is no such thing as a non-allergenic cosmetic, on the basis that almost any substance can, at least theoretically or potentially, trigger an allergy.

Many experts consider the term misleading, potentially lulling those with allergies into thinking a product is guaranteed to be safe for them.

The more scrupulous brands will use 'hypoallergenic' for products which exclude fragrances or known and common sensitizers such as MI / MCI. But others may use it more broadly and cynically, on the basis that most people will not react to their products or their ingredients (this goes for all cosmetics, given that over 50% of the population do not have allergies).

In the UK / EU, the 'hypoallergenic' term is likely to mean that the 26 fragrance allergens are absent from the product, and this will become a requirement from July 2019, when new guidance comes into effect calling for widely recognised skin sensitizers to be absent from any products labeled 'hypoallergenic'. This should also, then, apply to MI / MCI.

But always double check …

Meaningless marketing

There are other terms used by cosmetics companies which may be falsely reassuring to you.

Some examples:

- dermatologically tested
- formulated with families in mind
- gentle ingredients
- dermatologist approved
- sensitive / for sensitive skin
- skin kind
- natural / organic

Some of these statements or claims are meaningless in their own right, but with respect to MI allergy, they are generally irrelevant.

Of them, perhaps 'sensitive' is the most prevalent: there are dozens of examples of 'sensitive' products which *do* contain MI or MI / MCI on the market.

Don't be blindsided by them in your efforts to ascertain whether a product is safe for you. For that, you need to scrutinize ingredients, always.

Safe brands

The list of safe brands is ever-increasing, as many formulators look towards alternatives to the isothiazolinones.

That said, some formerly MI-free brands have been known to introduce a new product containing an isothiazolinone, so a safe brand today may not necessarily be a safe brand tomorrow.

Formulations also change — be they MI-free to MI-containing, or vice versa. And because old stock of previously unsafe products can remain on the shelf (or in an online shop) for many years, beware when buying a safely reformulated product that you're not buying the earlier, unsafe form.

Some global safe brands become well known to the isothiazolinone allergy community — such as Lush, and Body Shop — but there is a more comprehensive list on the Methylisothiazolinone Free website (www.mi-free.com).

Safe specific products

As for product types, the website has extensive listings which are kept up-to-date as much as possible, and are better sources of current information.

Try a search on the site, or use the drop-down menus for Cosmetics categories.

Some popular articles or listings, which you can easily search for, include:

- Listing of MI-free make-up;

- Article on hair dye / PPD-free hair dye;
- Collection of articles on MI-free hair care products.

Facebook is also a good source of personal recommendations from others with MI allergy. See Resources (page 95) for some suggested groups.

Zero-tolerance cosmetics

If you are highly sensitive to cosmetics ingredients and have a number of skincare issues, not least to the isothiazolinones, you may like to try a pure and minimalist cosmetic regimen, which excludes most or even all of the key culprits known to cause skin problems.

Although there is no hard evidence supporting their use in this circumstance, products with organic ingredients may be worth experimenting with, as isothiazolinones are sometimes used in pesticides more likely to be associated with non-organic farming practices.

The types of products you ought to look out for are very basic, single-ingredient or few-ingredient products such as raw or pure shea butter, and simple olive oil soaps.

Unscented Vaseline, although not considered 'natural' by most in the green beauty community, is non-reactive.

There's an article on the Allergy Insight website which lists a variety of low-allergen or (almost) no-allergen cosmetics which you may like to look into. It's called Allergen Free Skincare (www.allergy-insight.com/allergen-free-skincare).

Top tips

- Once you are diagnosed, you must go through your entire suite of cosmetics and toiletries, and those of others in the household, throughout the home, and give away or dispose of any that contain any of your allergens — without exception. A family member using MI-containing cosmetics can expose you to it through close contact. They very preferably ought to go MI-free too.

- Avoid buying cosmetics on the black market or from any temporary / street trader or traders overseas, who may be dealing in potentially stolen or counterfeit cosmetics. As tighter restrictions on MI and MCI kick in (in Europe, for example, but also in Canada and elsewhere), some manufacturers may be left with the prospect of either destroying excess, unsalable stock, or shifting it abroad to recoup some revenue. Watch out. It can, and does, end up anywhere.

- Given the lax regulations in the US, it is possible for amateur or start-up cosmetic formulators to produce and sell products very easily. Unless you can be 100% confident in their procedures and understanding, don't buy from very new or small brands, especially if they are unclear regarding ingredients.

- Lean away from water-based cosmetics towards oil-based formulations — such as body oils and body butters. Water-free cosmetics are far less likely to require preservation, and hence are likelier to be MI-free.

- It is good, general cosmetic practice to avoid keeping make-up and other cosmetics for many years. Actually *use* your (safe) cosmetics. Don't retain them for long periods, especially in warmer climates. The kinds of

'natural' products which often tend to be MI free will not usually last as long as conventional cosmetics, because the preservation system is likely to be gentler.
- Apply good cosmetic sense when travelling and staying in hotels. Take travel size packets and mini soaps by safe brands with you. Sample sizes are often readily available at beauty events and shows. (These are worth visiting for that purpose alone, but also so that you can freely enquire about ingredients and safety with brand representatives.) You can also decant some products, for instance shower gels, into smaller, sterilized bottles to take with you.

Legal limits

On one level, for those already diagnosed, the permitted maximum levels of isothiazolinone preservatives in cosmetics is irrelevant. They will need to avoid all products in which MI or MI / MCI are added ingredients, regardless of how much is present.

But others may be interested in the various regulations, official guidance and legal limits in their own and overseas territories, which may be useful for those travelling overseas.

Here is a brief summary, though bear in mind that laws are constantly being reviewed and updated.

- In the UK / EU, leave-on products such as moisturizers and mascara have to be isothiazolinone-free by law, but rinse-off products such as shampoo and shower gel can contain up to 15 parts per million (15ppm, or 0.0015%) of either MI or MI / MCI blend.
- In all non-EU countries, isothiazolinone preservatives are permitted in leave-on products, although some permit only MI, not the MI / MCI blend.

- In the US, cosmetics can contain up to 100ppm of MI, or 7.5ppm (leave-on) / 15ppm (rinse-off) of MI / MCI blend. These are recommended limits set out by the Cosmetic Ingredient Review (CIR).

- In Canada, 100ppm of MI is permitted in leave-on and rinse-off products, and 15ppm of MI / MCI blend is permitted in rinse-off products *only*.

- Many other nations, such as South Korea, Saudi Arabia, Brazil, Argentina and south east Asian countries, have rules in line with the Canadian ones.

- Most African nations have no set ppm limits at all.

In summary

- Watch out for methylisothiazolinone, methylchloroisothiazolinone or (outside UK / EU) Kathon CG on ingredient labels.

- Seek out recommendations from dedicated online resources or Facebook pages, but always double check ingredients with manufacturers as formulations can and do periodically change.

- If you are concerned about fragrance or parfum ingredients, especially in leave-on products, consult the manufacturer; if in doubt, it's safer to avoid.

- Don't be lulled into a false sense of security by 'greenwashing' or clever marketing terms such as 'eco friendly' or 'skin safe' or 'naturally derived' or 'organic'.

- Never buy or use anything which you can't confidently ascertain is MI free.

- Be aware of different rules when travelling overseas.

4. Home sense: safe household products

Many household products, particularly cleaning agents, such as laundry liquids, surface solutions and dishwashing detergents, contain isothiazolinone preservatives — not only MI and MCI, but benzisothiazolinone (BIT) and octylisothiazolinone (OIT), too.

Other products for the home where you may find the preservatives include air fresheners, fabric conditioners, anti-mold treatments, gardening products, wood polishes and many more besides.

They may also be present in pet care products, which are *not* classified as cosmetics, therefore not subject to cosmetic regulatory requirements, and therefore may contain higher concentrations of isothiazolinones than ordinarily encountered in equivalent products for humans.

Well over 90% of paints contain one or more of the isothiazolinone preservatives.

They may also be present in products such as glues, inks and arts supplies, including those for children.

It's a considerable problem.

It's a considerable problem even when you don't come into physical contact with the product, as you might with a dishwashing liquid.

Applied paint can off-gas isothiazolinone for over a month, causing symptoms.

Traces of isothiazolinones can be left behind on clothing and bedding in laundry, transferring to your skin and sustaining reactions.

Isothiazolinone-free household products are vital to your health. Don't be tempted to believe you can use gloves or other products such as face masks to fully protect yourself when using such products. They are only a partial help. Vaporized allergen and splashes of liquid will be your undoing.

Labeling

Labeling legislation for non-food and non-cosmetic products such as household detergents is not quite as strict, nor clear, and there may not be full disclosure of precise ingredients. This is especially true of product packaging — although some of the more considerate manufacturers will disclose more fully on their websites.

UK / EU labeling

That said, in the UK / EU, the presence of preservatives — including the isothiazolinones — *must* be declared in household cleaners, as must any of the 26 defined fragrance allergens, as well as any enzymes, disinfectants, and optical brighteners.

Major ingredients — such as surfactants, phosphates, bleaching agents, soaps and more — have to be declared within set percentage ranges, but only types or categories of these need to be listed: in other words, precisely named ingredients may not be given explicitly.

If for any reason you need them, you *may* find them on the product safety data sheets, which manufacturers should make available online, and these usually give a little more detail than provided on the product label.

Furthermore, there is a facility in the UK / EU where your medical service provider can request from manufacturers the full list of ingredients of any detergent, in order to explore health issues, including allergy, with you. Manufacturers are obliged to put contact details on their products from which this information can be requested. For piracy protection reasons, your medical professional is not permitted to pass on the full list of ingredients to you.

US labeling

In the US, products are regulated by the Consumer Product Safety Commission. The Household Products Labeling Act of 2009 proposed that ingredients should be declared on all cleaning products and detergent labels, including all fragrances, dyes and preservatives, but the bill was never enacted and 'died' in a previous congress.

This means that, essentially, manufacturers can disclose or not disclose ingredients.

Calling the brand's customer services helpline given on packaging may help, as might looking for a safety data sheet on the brand's website, but it is frustrating to have to go through this process, which has no guarantee of success in receiving a firm, trustworthy answer.

If and when you call a company, try to avoid sounding frustrated or demanding, as this will put some brands immediately on the defensive or else raise their suspicions. (Competitors sometimes call brands to try to obtain protected information.)

Instead, begin politely by explaining you have a severe allergy to isothiazolinone preservatives, are a potential customer who would like to use their products, and are calling to enquire whether they might be safe for you.

You may like to make clear that you are not looking for a complete list of ingredients, but for a confirmation that your trigger ingredients are absent from the product.

Be prepared to name and spell out each of the isothiazolinone preservatives.

It may be easier for a customer services operative to establish the safety of just one product, rather than the whole range of products by the brand, so specify its exact name if there is one in which you are particularly interested.

If you're told there's no mention of any isothiazolinone on the product's MSDS (material safety data sheet), politely point out that the ingredients listed there may not be exhaustive, and that you require greater reassurance.

If the brand assures you it is isothiazolinone-free after further investigation, and appears more open about disclosing its ingredients, you may like to ask which alternative preservatives are used instead, as this can be useful in establishing confidence in your query having been clearly understood.

Meaningless marketing

Again, as is the case with cosmetics, there are quite a lot of marketing terms manufacturers will use to convince you that their products are superior to those of competitors.

In terms of allergy safety, do not be reassured by the many you may see. These include:

- green and eco-friendly
- for a safe natural environment
- made to an organic formula
- gentle to your world
- plant-based cleaning solutions
- crafted with non-toxic ingredients

None of these, and the many others like them, imply that the product is isothiazolinone-free. Be wary of all.

There are also laundry products on the market, especially in the US, which claim to be 'hypoallergenic' and yet contain at least one isothiazolinone.

Another — sometimes seen on cosmetics too — is a 'chemical free' claim. This is nonsensical anyway: all formulations consist of chemicals. Laundry detergents, for example, are blends of ingredients such as water softeners, surfactants, optical brighteners, biological enzymes, fragrances, preservatives and other agents.

Chemicals are not to be feared — water is a chemical! — but no reassurance should be taken from a mistaken and potentially misleading 'chemical free' claim.

Safe products

Again, the Methylisothiazolinone Free website has extensive listings which are kept up-to-date as much as possible, and are better sources of current information. Input a search for your choice of product type or brand, or use the drop-down menu for the Household category.

Mirroring the situation with cosmetics, water-free formulations are far likelier to be safe.

For instance, dry laundry powder will probably be isothiazolinone-free, although there have been cases of products breaking this 'rule', albeit used in the hotel industry. Always check. A fragrance-free powder is likeliest to be the most 'allergy friendly' consumer option — in the US, those by Nellie's, Meliora and Molly's Suds are highly regarded, while in the UK, try Mangle & Wringer's.

Some brands are now improving their disclosure practices. S C Johnson, in particular, is worth a specific mention, as in December 2017 the company announced it had fulfilled a commitment to disclose the presence of 368 skin allergens on its ingredient website. The website, What's Inside S C Johnson (whatsinsidescjohnson.com), includes brands such as Glade, Pledge, Drano, Windex and more. Brands throughout dozens of countries are included, so you can search which particular products do and don't contain isothiazolinone ingredients.

Homemade products

For some people, a diagnosis of allergic contact dermatitis — to MI or other ingredient(s) — can be the push needed to look at making their own home cleaning and care products. This can help towards tackling indoor pollution, which in some can trigger respiratory aggravation, and also helps the environment. Naturally, this also eases any sensitivities.

In fact, some in the online allergy community strongly advise this home-made approach, at least at the beginning, when you may have to have a clearout of pre-manufactured products before establishing which you can and wish to use.

Baking soda (sodium bicarbonate), washing soda (sodium carbonate), castile soap (hard and/or liquid, but always fragrance free), white vinegar, lemons / lemon juice, borax, and essential oil drops (assuming you are not fragrance sensitive) are the ingredients to have in your armory if you wish to go down this road.

For instance, a customizable blend of fragrance-free liquid soap, baking soda and vinegar is a useful all-purpose cleaner, varying the proportions according to the job in hand. There are plenty of 'recipes' available online too. Some suggestions follow.

Toilet cleaner

For a simple freshen-up, use neat white vinegar, poured or squirted under rim, and then scrub, or spray on surfaces and wipe clean after a few minutes. For a more substantial clean, use half a cup of baking soda then add some vinegar to 'activate', and scrub as it does so.

Bathroom / shower cleaner

For a light clean, spray a mix of water and white vinegar in equal proportions, and wipe. For heavier grime, spray on pure white vinegar and rinse after an hour, or try baking soda blended with liquid castile soap.

Glass cleaner

Try white vinegar diluted with water; a drop of pure fragrance is optional.

Dishwashing liquid

Fragrance-free castile soap topped up with a little water, plus a little salt and vinegar.

Stain remover – for cookware / crockery

Salt mixed with a small amount of vinegar or lemon juice can clean and remove stains, although it can scratch some surfaces.

Surface cleaner

Again, water and vinegar in a 1:1 mix ratio (not suited to marble, granite or stone).

Oven cleaner

Spray warm oven with vinegar, then add salt or baking soda to trouble areas. Leave for a while, then wipe clean.

Washing powder

One grated Dr Bronner soap mixed with 250ml washing soda and 250ml borax. You can replace some or all of the borax with more washing soda. Use two tablespoons per load.

Fabric softener

Try a few tablespoons of white vinegar in the last rinse cycle.

Paints, varnishes, stains

Generally speaking, the various national or continental regulations for the labeling of domestic paints and related products are even less stringent than for detergents, and certainly than for cosmetics.

This compounds the already formidable problem when it comes to paints — which is that it is difficult to find MI-free varieties. All the major brands use isothiazolinones.

There *are* regulations, of course, and there are signs things are improving, although the situation is presently changeable. For instance, in the UK / EU, products with more than 0.1% MI must be labeled with an allergy warning, but this a very high limit and most unsafe paints do not contain anywhere near this quantity. The rule is under review, and a few manufacturers elect to declare their preservative ingredients voluntarily.

Powder paints, which you mix yourself, are usually safe, if you can find some.

It's easy to be misled by any paint claiming to be green, natural, non-toxic or asthma friendly, but this is no guarantee at all that it is isothiazolinone free.

The same applies to a paint which is low in or free of volatile organic compounds (VOCs). These are chemicals emitted as gases from liquids or solids, and some of which can cause detrimental health effects such as breathing issues in susceptible individuals.

Some brands which *are* either fully isothiazolinone-free or offer at least some isothiazolinone-free paints include Auro, Green Planet Paints and Renaissance Furniture Paint.

See the Paints directory on the Methylisothiazolinone Free site for more options (www.mi-free.com/household/methylisothiazolinone-free-paints).

Neutralizing solution

If you find yourself in a situation where the use of an unsafe paint is inevitable, some members of the Allergy to Isothiazolinone, Methylisothiazolinone and Benzisothiazolinone Facebook group have had success with a neutralizing wall wash applied to freshly applied (but dry) paint.

The recipe for the wash is a mix of 10% sodium bisulfite/bisulphite or sodium metabisulfite/metabisulphite to 90% water (ie dilute the active ingredient with nine times the quantity of water).

These sodium compounds are used in the brewing, winery and photography industries, so you should be able to buy the crystalline powder from, for instance, a brewery supply company.

It is unpleasantly pungent. Mixing with water will release sulphur / sulfur dioxide gas. If you are allergic to the gas, or to sulfites / sulphites, which are often used as food preservatives, and can cause breathing difficulties in a minority of people, you should avoid completely. Keep the compounds away from children.

Apply the solution as you would paint, although you may wish to test a small hidden patch initially to ensure it will not discolor. There may be a residue, but you should be able to later rinse it away.

This method is safe, but as a precaution open windows, wear a face mask (good practice anyhow when dealing with paint), and be sure *not* to use sodium bisulf*ate* / bisulph*ate*, which will not work.

5. Avoiding exposure

Once you've dealt with your cosmetics and your detergents, you'll have vastly improved the one environment you can exercise a high degree of control over — your home.

If you can convince friends and family to do likewise in their homes — great. This will help you considerably, and make their environment far safer for you when you visit or stay too.

What you have less control over, however, are other environments — such as public spaces and the workplace, for example.

What can you do?

Barrier methods

Avoidance is obviously the ideal, but there will be times when you're unable to be certain that the environment in which you find yourself will be free of your triggers, and so-called barrier methods — which put up a 'guard' against you and the outside world — may be helpful.

Topical barriers

Many people use moisturizers — including those specifically for eczema — as 'barrier' creams. These include Hydromol and Epaderm, for example.

As ordinary creams are absorbed by the skin, how well they act to 'shut out' any isothiazolinone you may touch — such as in a possibly unsafe detergent or from objects such as door handles or moving handrails — is uncertain, and likely to vary.

A product called Gloves in a Bottle, which is fragrance free, calls itself a shielding lotion and has good anecdotal reports from those with contact dermatitis.

Generally considered an excellent option is plain Vaseline.

Gloves

Finding safe gloves is a regular topic of discussion on the allergy support groups online, because the materials used in glove manufacture are sometimes treated with isothiazolinone-containing disinfectants or finishing solutions, and it can be difficult to get a definitive answer from manufacturers on processes and ingredients used.

Plain white cotton gloves or cotton liner gloves — washed several times in MI-free laundry detergent and rinsed thoroughly — are a good bet for everyday 'dry' protection. They are widely available. Close-fitting ones can act as 'liner' gloves, inside a pair of protective gloves, which offer the added advantage that hands won't get as sweaty or sticky.

But which protective gloves?

The consensus among the community appears to be to avoid latex gloves, because isothiazolinones are used to preserve many of the emulsions from which latex gloves are made, and it seems that this may be the case for PVC / vinyl gloves too.

Furthermore, a 2014 case report published in the journal *Contact Dermatitis* suggested that natural rubber gloves "might not protect against skin penetration of methylisothiazolinone".

So what might be safe?

<u>Nitrile gloves</u>

Some people — but not all — report success with nitrile gloves.

Nitrile is a synthetic rubber and is a more impenetrable material than some others used by glove manufacturers.

Some gloves have powder added, which helps when putting them on. Normally, this is plain corn starch, but there is a concern that this can absorb the materials used in gloves, including allergens such as latex and others, and then disperse them in the atmosphere when the gloves are removed, risking the health of an allergic individual.

Some gloves have chemical 'accelerators' added during manufacture. These help provide stretch, add strength, and increase durability and stability of the glove. The main classes of chemicals used as accelerators are thiurams, (dithio)carbomates, and mercaptobenzothiazoles — which are not isothiazolinones, despite the similarity in name. These chemical accelerators can, however, cause or facilitate type IV contact allergies.

The solution, then, albeit not a 100% guaranteed safe one, is to look for accelerator-free and powder-free nitrile gloves, of which there are a number of suppliers online, usually selling in boxes of 100. Many will be marked as allergy safe or 'hypoallergenic'.

Be wary of any gloves advertising themselves as anti-microbial or having an anti-bacterial coating as they may have been treated with chemicals whose make-up it could be difficult to establish.

Colored nitrile gloves are useful, as any breakages are more easily spotted than in white or flesh-colored gloves.

Read instructions carefully as some gloves should not be used with certain chemicals, such as oxidisers or strong acids.

Brands you may like to look at include:

- Vitrex (UK; www.vitrex.co.uk)

- Unigloves (UK; www.unigloves.co.uk — look for their Zero gloves)
- Eagle (US; www.eagleprotect.com — they have 'Sensitive' Nitrile Gloves)
- Ansell (US; www.ansell.com — they have MICROTOUCH® nitrile gloves with 'advanced allergy prevention').

There are many more which you can find through an online search.

Disposable gloves can be particularly useful, incidentally, if you work in a profession in which you are otherwise required to wash your hands multiple times a day — for instance, catering or nursing.

Clothing

It is tempting in summer to expose more skin, but think ahead about your plans for the day and with what your skin may come into direct contact.

Wearing shorts or a skirt on public transport may mean the backs of your legs rub against plastic or leather seating. If that seating has been cleaned with a risky detergent or had a fabric coating applied to it, or else previously come into contact with the skin of other passengers who have used unsafe cosmetics, then this could irritate your skin.

Light, airy clothes, which cover up skin, may be the better option.

Protective clothing

Research shows that off-gas emitted from recently applied paint can trigger skin sensitivities directly, so close-fitting, tight-weave clothing may offer some protection in a situation where you may be exposed.

Facial masks

Facial allergy masks tend to focus on filtering particulates — pollens and pollutant particulates, for example.

However, to have any hope of dealing with chemicals such as isothiazolinones or fragrances or other volatile organic compounds (VOCs) that can off-gas from paint, for instance, then chemical filters made from carbon are required.

The Respro® Allergy Mask comes with a particle filter but can be purchased with an additional combination chemical/particle filter that includes a Dynamic Activated Charcoal Cloth (DACC™) to adsorb dozens of chemicals.

It's important to stress that its manufacturers have said that they have *not* tested the product's effectiveness on the isothiazolinones, but they say "in all probability, owing to its molecular make up, it will be adsorbed if present in an airborne environment. Methylisothiazolinone is a hydrocarbon and DACC is very good for the adsorption of hydrocarbons".

Although avoidance is always the best approach, such masks may be useful for when you find yourself in an unavoidable situation, such as having to walk through a recently painted public area.

To find out more, see the Respro website at www.respro.com. They deliver worldwide.

There is a full-length article on allergy face masks, which may also interest you, featuring both Respro and several other options, at www.mi-free.com.

Goggles

These may also help as a temporary measure in any environment where there may be steam or heat or aerosolized or vaporized chemical particles.

You may like to put some Vaseline onto the rims where contact with your face is made — swimmers often do this to ensure a closer seal and increase comfort.

Air purifiers / filters

Perhaps not 'barrier' methods, per se, as these aim to remove the threat from your environment rather than merely blocking it from entering your system, but still relevant.

That said, there is limited information on this method of self-protection. Particulate filters, such as HEPA (high efficiency particulate air / absorber) filters, designed to trap dust, pollen and mold, are not able to trap (small) isothiazolinone molecules, but they may help with unrelated allergies such as hay fever, and therefore 'ease' the pressure on your immune system.

Although the picture is unclear, it's probably safe to assume that only carbon-enabled purifiers, with activated charcoal filters to adsorb volatile organic compounds, are worth trying as far as the isothiazolinones are concerned.

There are some anecdotal reports of these working well, but there appears to be no published research, and manufacturers seem reluctant to make claims about specific chemicals, typically restricting themselves to general ones that they 'help to adsorb VOCs' or some such.

There are plenty of air filters available which utilize both HEPA and activated carbon technologies, and these may be the best options to begin with. (HEPA treated air is required for the carbon filtration to work, so both are needed.)

IQAir (www.iqair.com) is a reputable brand, recommended by some people with isothiazolinone allergy.

A more 'belt and braces' approach may be to choose an air purifier with both of the above — plus zeolite. Zeolite is a porous mineral made up of silicon compounds, aluminium and oxygen, which is claimed by some to be better able to trap small-molecular gases such as formaldehyde, ammonia and carbon monoxide.

Several filters by Austin (www.austinair.com) use a combined carbon-zeolite extraction medium, including the Healthmate Plus.

For more suggestions and what to consider when buying a filter or purifier for allergies, there is an article on Allergy Insight (www.allergy-insight.com/air-filters-and-purifiers) which may be useful.

A note about ionizers or combined purifier-ionizers: these are probably best avoided. They charge airborne particles, which then become attracted to walls and ceilings, adhering to them. They may be useful to protect against molds and bacteria, but don't help tackle polluting VOCs, and may generate internal ozone, which is harmful in itself, but also may increase the natural levels of formaldehyde.

Your working environment

The potential for exposure may be considerable at your place of work.

If the building you work in is being redecorated, the paint is likely to be a hazard.

If it's air conditioned, the cleaning agents used in the air conditioning system are likely to be isothiazolinone-containing, meaning it could end up in the internal atmosphere

— doubly so if air fresheners are used too, as these aren't always safe either.

The office cleaners are likely to use surface wipes or polish which could be triggering.

There will be further potential reactions in products used in the restrooms and any shared kitchen facilities.

Sadly, some people — such as painters, hair stylists, massage therapists and decorators — have found they have had to relinquish their jobs or careers due to their allergies.

It's worth speaking to your line manager or human resources department about your situation. Another key reason to ensure that you have a firm diagnosis, with a letter from medical professionals, is that it serves as evidence to support your case and ensure senior colleagues take your situation seriously. There may be actions which can be taken. Isothiazolinone-free products are now readily available, and detergents and other materials can be found even for offices, in the bulk amounts often required, in order to replace any unsafe ones. Good employers will listen and try to accommodate your requirements. They have a duty of care.

Printer inks can be preserved with isothiazolinones. Printers and photocopiers are warm, and vaporized ink can cause symptoms in this environment. Take care with handling freshly printed copies and if your desk is situated near a printer in the office, consider asking whether you can sit elsewhere, or whether the printer can be relocated.

You may be at risk if you're a hairdresser or work in the beauty industry, or in engineering or mechanics, or the medical industry, and many others. Barrier methods such as gloves and masks may help, but are unlikely to be a convenient or practical solution for all, sadly.

School

Similar precautions apply, if your child has allergies.

School principals and teachers will be used to holding conversations on this subject with other parents, given so many children have food allergies and other sensitivities these days, so don't be apprehensive.

It can help to formalize the care children receive at school through an Individual Health Plan, signed off and agreed to by all parties. An IHP outlines, for example, the precautions which must be taken to manage the child's allergy, where any medication will be stocked, and the responsibilities of parents, the student, the school nurse, teachers and the head principal. The IHP should be reviewed annually, at least, and it may require the support and consultation of your doctor or dermatologist. Your national eczema charity (see Resources on page 95) should be able to advise and help, if you need guidance.

Particular considerations include school art supplies such as paints, glues, clays, and inks. Jill Sandager, mother to a young MI-allergic daughter, blogs at The Snarky Dabbler, and has addressed this issue in a regularly updated post (snarkydabbler.blogspot.com/2016/08/methylisothiazolinone-and-school.html), which has lots of safe / probably safe suggestions.

Do take extreme care with products such as toy 'slime' which is water based, sticky and may well contain isothiazolinones.

Powder-free nitrile gloves for children are available. Search online.

Driving / public transport

As already mentioned, clothing protection can help to some degree.

Leathers and other upholstery materials may be treated with potentially problematic chemicals, so prolonged exposure could irritate you.

Bare hands on a new leather steering wheel might be risky. Wear cotton driving gloves or use a washable steering wheel cover.

Bear in mind that if you take your car for servicing or detailing, isothiazolinone-containing detergents or polishes may well be used, not only on visible or obvious areas, but potentially in places such as the air-conditioning systems. Ask your valet to refrain, or offer safe product suggestions, or as an absolute last resort let your car 'air' for as long as possible and later wipe surfaces with a plain damp cloth or safe natural solution.

Isothiazolinones are used in diesel production, incidentally, which is something to be aware of, although perhaps principally relevant only to mechanics or service station personnel. Always wash hands after pumping fuel, or preferably wear gloves, and consider wearing a face mask when you visit a service station.

Medical / hospital treatment

It may seem perverse that the risk of inadvertent exposure when you're at your surgery, clinic or hospital is high — but high it is.

Matters have improved — safer medical gloves, for instance, as outlined previously — but there remain plenty of potential traps in medical settings.

Make sure all your medical records state that you have isothiazolinone allergy — medical service providers often use shared medical databases — and that every consultant or member of medical staff you meet is informed or reminded verbally.

Hand sanitizer should now be safe in the UK / EU, but not necessarily elsewhere. Avoid using it unless you are certain of the brand, and offer to wash hands with your own liquid soap if needs be. MI-free brand Dr Bronner offers convenient small bottles.

You *have* to check anything that might come into contact with you. Make it a habit even when it may just be pure alcohol. So, if you're receiving an injection, ask the nurse to check with what the needle was sterilized and to verify the swab is safe.

Wound dressings have been found to contain isothiazolinone preservatives, so ask these to be checked. Ditto any type of adhesive or plaster.

The same applies to any gloves the practitioner is wearing to examine you.

If you are to lie down on a couch, you may prefer to bring your own towel or sheet, which you know is safely washed, especially if you are required to undress.

Ultrasound gel, *not* classified as a cosmetic, is a particular problem, although some MI-free gels are available. In the US, the Clear Image brand and some Aquasonic products (eg Aquasonic 100) are safe, but you may need to check for other allergens. Lubricant gels, as used in Pap or cervical smears, must also be checked.

Oral medication should be safe, but note that the antibiotic metronidazole has a documented potential cross-reaction to isothiazolinone preservatives. Play safe and refuse to be prescribed it, should the situation arise.

You also need to check with your dentist or his or her dental assistant about mouthwash, oral disinfectant and the materials used to sterilize equipment.

Ditto any eye drops from an optometrist.

Bars / restaurants

There is a possibility that unsafe surface wipes or dishwashing detergents are used here, meaning potential exposure to trace quantities through glassware, crockery, utensils and table-tops, for instance.

This is a tricky one. You can minimize risk by, for example, drinking beer from a bottle rather than a glass, and by bringing your own essential items, such as cutlery and paper napkins, or using your own recyclable coffee cup, or else by enquiring in advance which brands of detergents the food outlet uses.

That said, some find they don't react to these trace exposures.

Vacations / hotels

Bear in mind that hoteliers and travel agents are increasingly used to receiving and accommodating allergy-related requests, so don't be shy of making your requirements known in advance, and do as much pre-planning as you can.

Many establishments advertise themselves as 'allergy aware'. Call ahead and ask for 'no towels' and to remove any air freshener in the room, for example.

You may need to bring your own sheets, pillow slip and towels. An alternative option is to use a sleeping bag liner or sleep sack in bed. Bring products with distinctive patterns /

designs so that they are not accidentally mistaken for the hotel's own and removed by staff.

In your living quarters, avoid going barefoot on floors which may have been cleaned with an MI-containing detergent or carpet cleaner.

Consider a barrier cream before using any swimming pools. Use flip-flops to protect feet, and wear goggles always. Although the water's sterilizing chemicals are unlikely to be MI-containing, there's a chance that sun cream worn by other swimmers could wash off into the water to enough of a degree to trigger a reaction, especially when it is busy. Note that sun cream in the EU should now be safe; that said, overseas visitors or tourists may well be using non-EU products or brands ...

You may want to clean with your own products or an all-purpose cleaner — bring gloves if you intend to do so.

An air purifier might help. Air conditioner systems in hotels are often cleaned with MI-containing detergents, so off-gas can circulate in the air. If you can't use a purifier, ask if the air conditioning can be switched off, and make use of a simple electric fan.

Skin / beauty / hair treatment

It goes without saying that before any form of beauty or hair treatment, at any establishment, you must check with your beautician, therapist or hairdresser that the cosmetics she or he plans on using on you are safe.

This will need to be undertaken in advance of your appointment, and you must be rigorous in double-checking everything on the day.

Isothiazolinones are found in a significant proportion of professional nail care and hair care products, including shampoos, conditioners, styling products and manicure products.

The same goes for eyebrow microblading — or indeed any tattoos. A Swiss study found that almost a quarter of tattoo inks contain benzisothiazolinone, and one in 14 contained formaldehyde. Dyes can contain other contact allergens: blue ink tends to contain cobalt, for example. If you can't be certain that dyes are free from your contact allergens, then do not allow yourself to be tattooed.

Clothing

Again, there is an absence of research, but several with MI allergy report itch and other reactions when wearing or after trying on new clothing.

Launder new clothing and tread cautiously with leather shoes, belts and other goods, including watch straps.

When trying on clothing in a store it may help to wear tight-fitting eczema cotton clothing underneath.

Also take care with going barefoot in new shoes, not only due to the materials themselves, but to the glues used, for example, to fix insoles. Symptoms can be unpleasant if feet get sweaty, creating a humid atmosphere conducive to reactions.

If using a dry cleaning service, ask about the agents the assistants plan to use on your clothing. Pure steam cleaning may be the best option.

There have also been reports of reactions to new spectacle frames.

Home furnishing

Many report reactions to newly acquired materials and products for the home, such as mattresses, bedding, upholstery, furniture, curtains, carpets and more.

Hampering your efforts to stay safe is the fact that there is no way to remove isothiazolinones from non-washable materials, so 'barrier' methods may be the only counter-measure you can take. It is probable that over time trace isothiazolinones will off-gas, but this may feel like small consolation if you react soon after acquiring the new items.

Cover new or relatively new leather seating with safe blankets.

Be very wary of any fabrics or materials treated to be anti-microbial or anti-dust mite.

Avoid walking barefoot on new rugs or carpeting.

Furniture which is kept in storage for a long time by manufacturers may require an anti-microbial treatment to protect surfaces. IKEA, for instance, are known to use isothiazolinone-containing compounds to treat and preserve their products. Self-assembly furniture, stored in boxes and plastic wrappings, may be more problematic as off-gasing is hindered. Consider scrubbing it down and allowing it to air before you assemble or use.

In summary ...

It's impossible to list all potential situations in which you may be exposed, and this chapter has only given you a selection of them. There's also potential exposure at the gym — all those shared machines (safe wipes can be a godsend here), and cosmetics in the humid shower rooms — and without doubt you'll be able to think of many others.

Although you'll have appreciated that vigilance is required, hyper-vigilance can be stressful and counter-productive. Sensitivities vary, and those more mildly affected will not be troubled by some of the potential exposures described in this chapter.

Despite the difficulties and precautions you may need to take, try to retain a sense of calm and perspective and don't fear every single external potential contact. Some mistakes or minor inadvertent exposures are inevitable, and you will learn from them. Taking the advice given will protect you against the worst, and you will learn quickly how best to safeguard your wellbeing in the long run.

6. Skin health, skin reactions

Post-diagnosis, you may be feeling overwhelmed with the prospect of the changes you have to make. This is understandable. We will be looking at emotional issues in chapter 8, but in this one we look at physical health issues — getting well and staying that way.

You may have long-standing troubled skin, be it mild or severe, due to ongoing exposure to the isothiazolinones and perhaps other allergens. Your consultants will be best placed to advise, in either case. Avoidance of triggers is obviously key, and hopefully the advice in the previous chapters will help.

In an ideal world, as soon as you've been diagnosed and set about undertaking avoidance tactics, all will resolve.

But, sadly, we don't live in an ideal world …

Medication

Medication may be required and prescribed to you — both to address long-standing problems that preceded your diagnosis, and the occasional ones which may manifest due to accidental exposure.

Anti-histamines

These counteract the inflammatory histamine that may be released in your body due to exposure to allergen(s).

That said, MI allergy is a type IV reaction, in which histamine release in the body is not involved.

Some people with MI allergy also use a low daily dose of antihistamine as a preventative, or to help them sleep if their skin is in an uncomfortable state, but whether or not this is actually effective is uncertain, and you should always consult a specialist before commencing.

Zyrtec (cetirizine) or Benadryl (diphenhydramine) for nighttime use and Tagamet (cimetidine), Allegra (fexofenadine) and Claritin (loratadine) for morning might be appropriate in some circumstances, mainly if you have other allergies.

Topical cortisone / corticosteroids

A topical cortisone or corticosteroid to apply to your skin — such as Novasone (mometasone furoate), Dermovate (clobetasol propionate), or Cloderm (clocortolone pivalate) — may also be recommended.

These can come in various strengths and forms.

Inexplicably, some steroid *creams* and *lotions* can contain MI, so ensure checks are undertaken before accepting the prescription.

Steroid *ointments* aren't usually affected, but still check.

Use only as directed and *never* over-apply.

Topical steroids can thin skin when used for extended periods.

Immuno-modulators

Other topical ointments which may be suggested are Protopic (tacrolimus monohydrate) or Elidel (pimecrolimus), which are immuno-modulators, helping to decrease the immune-related inflammatory reaction in the skin.

Again, these should be only used as directed and sparingly.

Systemic corticosteroids

More serious or extensive dermatitis may require systemic corticosteroids — such as Prednisone — taken (orally) for a period of a week or less.

There is some concern over their use, however, as there can be cumulative harm from multiple short courses, such as an increased risk of osteoporosis, long-term, so this is not a course to be taken lightly.

They also dull the immune system and can cause short-term neurological side-effects.

Immuno-suppressants

These drugs are less likely to be prescribed, but in some circumstances might be. They slow down the production of new immune cells, thereby reducing inflammation.

Methotrexate is one such drug. It is taken in very small, occasional doses, and can take several weeks to have any effect.

Antibiotics

If skin is infected, they may be prescribed.

As always, complete the course if you need to take them.

Phototherapy / light therapy

PUVA (psoralen and ultraviolet A) therapy is a treatment for problem skin, albeit usually for psoriasis.

Psoralen is a naturally occurring drug which can be taken orally or applied to the skin. As it is so good at absorbing UV, exposing the skin to small doses of light can have a therapeutic effect, although it will not suit all people with MI allergy and related chronic skin problems. It tends to be used when there is longer-standing damage caused by ongoing issues. There are also some possible side effects — increased photo-sensitivity, nausea, itchy skin and more.

Some dermatologists may just recommend you expose problem skin to the sun for roughly ten minutes either early or late in the day (not around midday or early afternoon).

Cosmetics

It is generally advised you avoid soaps — these are alkaline and strip the skin's protective barrier — and instead use pH-balanced cleansers for sensitive skin, which should not leave your skin dry or vulnerable. Derma E's Sensitive Skin Cleanser is one such product.

A moisturizer or emollient will help. Outside UK / Europe especially, check that any you use are isothiazolinone free.

Ointments tend to be the oiliest, the richest, and the most effective at retaining moisture into the skin; creams are a middle-ground option; lotions are wetter and less oily, and usually less effective. Depending on your symptoms and your skin's dryness, your consultant will recommend one or more.

Inflamed skin tends to suit cream or lotion; dry but non-inflamed skin may be better with ointment-type products.

Don't massage or rub in emollients vigorously: use in appropriate quantities, as indicated, and smooth in gently, regularly, perhaps after washing.

Some emollients can be used as cleansers or bath soaks too, but seek guidance.

Therapeutic bathing

Some with MI allergy or other allergic contact dermatitis / eczema swear by different kinds of baths — both while they're in recovery post-diagnosis, and to maintain skin health on an ongoing basis.

The key in all cases is to not have the water too hot. It should *never* scald.

For an ordinary everyday bath, the 'soak and seal' approach is useful, because it helps hydrate dry and irritated skin. It basically consists of a lukewarm bath lasting no longer than ten minutes, using an ultra-gentle detergent (no strong scrubbing), followed by a gentle patting dry of the skin with a clean towel — so that it retains some 'dampness' — followed by sufficient emollient.

There are also some tailored therapeutic approaches that may be appropriate.

Bleach baths

These are not as scary as they may sound, and seem popular, though it is vital you speak to your doctor before attempting one, and that you ensure you know exactly what you are doing.

Do *not* try bleach baths without getting medical clearance. If you have very dry skin they may be uncomfortable and unsuitable. They may not be recommended for very young children either. If you have asthma, and bleach aggravates your breathing, it's best to avoid them. Open or bleeding skin should *not* be exposed to diluted bleach, and *never* expose any skin at all to undiluted bleach.

Bleach is essentially a solution of sodium hypochlorite. Diluted bleach baths help kill bacteria such as *staphylococcus aureus* on the skin, and this helps to not only reduce inflammation, but lower the risk of skin infections following any severe flare-up.

Several eczema organisations provide guidance on their websites for bleach baths, so you may like to follow, for instance, your national charity's recommendations. (See Resources on page 95.)

Dilution is, obviously, essential. Be extremely careful with your dosages.

First, make sure the tub is fully rinsed and clean, and then draw your usual quantity of water into the bath.

Use plain household bleach (of around 5% sodium hypochlorite) *not* concentrated bleach (which is around 8% sodium hypochlorite). Around half a cup of household bleach mixed thoroughly into a full standard bathtub of water is the usual recommendation, but you may like to start with a third of a cup. Also use considerably less if you tend to take shallower baths — around a quarter of a cup of bleach into half a bathtub of water is about right. Do not add anything else to the tub.

For younger children, provided your doctor or dermatologist has approved the treatment, around one teaspoon of household bleach per gallon of water is what the American Academy of Dermatology suggest.

Although they should not contain any isothiazolinone, always check. Many household bleaches do contain soap and perfume, though, which may cause irritation. Try to find one without. Sometimes 'value' or thin bleaches may be appropriate, but check ingredients and concentrations carefully, and consider asking your doctor for recommendations, especially if you are uncertain about ingredients (which may not always be fully disclosed) and quantities.

In the UK, you can instead use Milton Sterilising Fluid, which is 2% sodium hypochlorite, and which is free of other additives. As it is weaker than household bleach, you'll need more. A cupful for a full standard bathtub is about right, but again scale down for shallower baths, and for children.

Time your soak, and take care *not* to doze. Soak for at least five minutes, but *not* more than ten minutes maximum, keeping the head, and especially eyes, well away from the water. Do not 'wash', or use any detergent, soap, shampoo or oil. This is a soak, remember. Rinse off fully with warm water afterwards. Pat skin dry. Then moisturize.

Repeat weekly, or at most twice-weekly, or as advised by your doctor, or as determined by your skin's condition and any improvement.

If you experience any discomfort or reaction, discontinue with the baths and speak to your doctor or dermatologist at once.

A reminder: take extreme care with bleach baths. If you're nervous or uncertain about them, avoid them, and perhaps try one of the other options in this section.

Vinegar baths

Another anti-bacterial approach. Try a cup of vinegar in a shallow bath or several cups for a fuller bath, following the same approach as per a bleach bath. Avoid any 'flavored' vinegars. Apple cider vinegar has a good reputation. Rinse, pat, moisturize.

Oatmeal baths

Colloidal oatmeal is best. This is finely ground oats, which exposes and releases more of the active ingredients within oats, helping them to disperse better in bathwater.

Oats have a long history of therapeutic use in skincare — witness their inclusion in many emollients — and there appear to be several reasons: they contain anti-inflammatory avenathramide compounds, hydrating and water-retaining beta-glucans, and cleansing natural saponin chemicals.

You can make your own colloidal oats by using a blender to grind 100% pure oats into a fine powder which dissolves fully in water, producing a 'milk'. Use a cupful for a full bath; much less for younger children in shallower baths. Due to a small risk of sensitization to oats, don't consider bathing children in oats before they have been introduced safely into the diet, and are tolerated.

Longer soaks are permitted with oatmeal — around a quarter of an hour is good. You can rinse a little if your skin feels sticky, and beware that the bath may be slippery. Then, as ever, moisturize.

Saltwater baths

This can help inflammation or sting. Ordinary table or sea salt is fine. Epsom salts which aren't fragranced are good too. Use around a cup for a half bathtub of water.

Managing flare-ups

Despite your best intentions and precautions, there may be occasions when previously healed skin flares up once again, or you go through a literal 'bad patch' when reactions appear to be more regular and your skin won't settle.

The return of symptoms can suggest a recent inadvertent isothiazolinone exposure, but may also be down to other factors — such as other allergies, or even changes in the environment.

You may get reactions manifesting not at the point of contact with the allergen, but at the original site where you were sensitized and first experienced reactions before diagnosis. For many with MI allergy, those sites are quite often either the hands or the eyes. Were you originally sensitized through mascara and later exposed yourself to washing up liquid with MI in it? You may have felt your eyelids stinging, even if you touched the liquid with only your hands.

Try to find out the cause, if you think it was something with which you came into contact:

- Has someone in your life changed his or her fragrance?
- Are you sure none of the products you are using have new or updated formulations?
- Did you visit someplace new?
- Have your offices been redecorated, or have your employers switched their detergent suppliers?

Your detective skills will certainly have to improve when you become allergic to isothiazolinones!

If you can't identify a cause or source, it may be worth discussing the problem with your dermatologist or immunologist. It could be a new allergy.

Some of the recommendations and treatments given earlier should help you. Aquaphor Healing Ointment is one product which many in the MI allergy community appear to turn to for flared-up skin. Another is Hydromol Ointment.

If you prefer to keep things 'natural', pure organic coconut oil may be worth a try. Or else SkinSmart Antimicrobial (www.skinsmartantimicrobial.com), which is a water-based dilution of salt and hypochlorous, endorsed by the National

Eczema Association, which promotes healing and helps soothe raw and irritated skin.

Consider every slip-up a learning experience, and forgive yourself. Mistakes happen. And you will get much better at avoidance and skin-health maintenance.

Diet and the skin

This is not a book about diet, nutrition, nor 'wellness'.

However, it's important to touch upon these subjects, because so much is written and spoken about them that they loom large over everybody who has to give more consideration to their health than others might.

There is some research on diet and eczema, but it is not yet conclusive. Those with forms of eczema are likelier to be sensitive to allergens such as milk, gluten, eggs and others than those without eczema, but they are still unlikely to be so from a purely statistical standpoint, and it's generally considered unwise to remove these staple foods from your diet without a firm medical diagnosis, or at the very least without guidance from a registered dietitian (RD), certainly in the case of children's diets.

There is modest evidence to suggest that a so-called anti-inflammatory diet, which includes oily fish, nuts, olive oil, colorful vegetables, fruit and spices, may be helpful, all the while keeping intake of saturated fat, sugar and highly processed foods quite low.

Probiotic-rich foods — such as yoghurt, sauerkraut, kefir, miso and other 'live' or fermented products — are increasingly being recognised as healthful to the gut, which may well have a knock-on effect on the skin and other parts of the body.

If you follow a restricted diet — be it due to veganism or coeliac disease (gluten hypersensitivity) or any other — then input and guidance from an RD is essential.

Ethical or medical diets are one thing, but please avoid obvious fads, such as any form of paleo diet, for which there is no supporting evidence, nor indeed any logical argument: humans evolved to eat a wide omnivorous diet, so aim for just that as much as you can, within your own ethical, allergy or religious boundaries.

Really, the best approach is to not worry too much about food.

Instead: cook, enjoy what you eat, do it in the company of people you care about, only take dietary advice from those truly qualified to give it to you, not from those who reveal their midriffs on social media platforms, and *never* assume you can substitute supplements for a rounded diet.

7. Other allergies

Sadly, isothiazolinone allergies don't necessarily occur in isolation, and often come partnered with other allergies, which you or your child may have been diagnosed with via patch testing at the same time — or which may develop at a later date.

Fragrance allergies

Allergies to the isothiazolinones and to fragrances are significantly associated, meaning if you react to one or more in either category, you're statistically likelier to have an allergy to one or more in the other.

In chapter 3, we considered the possibility of reacting to a fragrance ingredient preserved with an isothiazolinone and then later used in the manufacture of another cosmetic.

Those with MI allergy who react to cosmetics often suspect 'hidden' traces of isothiazolinone in fragrance ingredients, but statistically it is more likely to be a distinct allergy to one or more fragrance compounds, and this can be diagnosed through patch testing.

You may instinctively feel that you react to fragrances and may opt for 'fragrance free' without a formal diagnosis, managing your skin reactions accordingly. If you're happy and that works for you — great.

In fact, there appears to be a growing movement against fragrance in society, given its allergic and health impact, including its potentially severe effects on many who have asthma. This growing 'discent' is gathering pace, and many are moving away from perfumed lifestyles.

Either way, beware of using any fragranced products on broken skin, as this can make you more susceptible to developing new allergies.

That said, there is a persistent myth, however, that if you *do* have fragrance allergies, you necessarily need to avoid *all* fragrances.

Actually, this is unlikely. And this is another reason why patch testing is so useful: it can pinpoint not only MI / MCI allergies, but help identify other allergies too — although when it comes to fragrances, there are some limitations.

The fragrance allergens

Limitations are inevitable because there are thousands of fragrance components or molecules in cosmetics and household products, and it is impossible to test each one individually through patch testing, in order to pinpoint precisely which elements you may be reacting to.

Many of these are at least theoretically capable of triggering reactions, and all occur in varying combinations in hundreds of natural extracts, oils, blends and synthetic perfumes.

And don't be fooled into assuming that natural fragrances are less likely to trigger allergies than synthetic fragrances. This is another myth. If anything, it's the other way around. Never look upon 'natural' or 'healing' essential oils or fragrance compounds as 'safe'. Artificial options may actually be better from an allergy perspective.

Some fragrance components, then, are more likely to trigger allergies than others. Because of this variation in allergenic potential, only those riskier fragrance compounds are likely to be tested routinely on patch testing panels, and some will be blended together in standard mixes. These go by the names Fragrance Mix I and Fragrance Mix II. Other fragrance compounds can sometimes be additionally tested individually.

If you have tested positive to mix I or II, it means you are allergic to at least one fragrance compound, but possibly more than one, and if the compound is naturally occurring, then you will also be allergic to the oils in which it is found. The more you react to, the more complex management becomes — unless of course you opt for a strict fragrance-free regimen.

Names and labeling

In the UK / EU, there are 26 fragrance allergens which have to be explicitly named in ingredients lists when present in cosmetics above certain levels. You will normally find them at the very end, after the preservatives. Among them are geraniol, eugenol, cinnamal, limonene, linalool, benzyl alcohol, farnesol and coumarin, and some of these are included in the I and II mixes.

Your dermatologist should be able to give you the names of these, and any essential oils or popular fragrances in which they occur. If not, ask.

Elsewhere, including in North America, fragrances can far more easily 'hide' within products. Some brands, in seeking to protect their trade secrets, will not tell you which components make up their fragrances, and may describe them merely as 'parfum' on the label.

If you call their customer helplines, they may concede to giving 'yes' or 'no' answers regarding specific oils or fragrances. Some will be more helpful than others.

If essential oils are added, these should be declared in name.

No fragrance, low fragrance ...

Some oils are less likely to trigger allergies due to being free from or extremely low in the 26 European fragrance allergens. These include myrrh, vetiver, sandalwood, cedarwood and patchouli. A cautious trial and error approach may work for you, or you could look for a fragrance blended specifically to be low allergen, although there can never be guarantees.

Alternatively, you could just use non-fragrance ingredients which you happen to like the smell of — for instance, coconut.

A final point: remember too that neither 'scent free' nor 'fragrance free' necessarily indicates products free of fragrance compounds — these terms may just indicate that the manufacturer is claiming that the products have little aroma. Masking fragrance may have been used, in order to cover up the possibly unpleasant or undesirable aromas of other ingredients.

Many cosmetics companies include at least a few fragrance-free products within their range, but brands which are entirely fragrance free are few.

Cosmetic brands which offer some (or only) fragrance-free products include: Vanicream, Free & Clear, QV Skincare, Green People (the Scent Free range), and JASON No Scent / Fragrance Free.

Household brands which offer some (or only) fragrance-free products include: Earthview, Meliora, Bio-D, Attitude and Surcare.

Allergy to formaldehyde

Formaldehyde and compounds which release formaldehyde are preservatives widely used in cosmetics, detergents, paints and in various industries, especially the clothing industry (new clothes can be sources of exposure) and textile industry.

The name formaldehyde causes concern among some people, but this is generally needless. It is a natural gas, produced in our bodies, and essential for some biochemical processes within it.

It is naturally present within some foods too. Pears are high in formaldehyde, for example. According to informational database CosmeticsInfo.org, the amount released by a formaldehyde-preserved shampoo in a single wash is equivalent to that found in one pear.

So formaldehyde is likely to be a concern only if you are sensitive to it. As with fragrances, formaldehyde allergies and isothiazolinone allergies are associated. This exacerbates the difficulty for those allergic to both — especially if you have concerns about parabens, another class of preservatives, making your choice even more limited.

Inconveniently, the names of formaldehyde-releasing preservatives don't include 'formaldehyde', so those allergic to them need to memorize them.

Methylene glycol / methanediol is hydrated formaldehyde.

Here is a list of the main formaldehyde releasers / formaldehyde donors:

- quaternium-15
- 2-bromo-2-nitropropane-1,3 diol (Bronopol)
- diazolidinyl urea
- imidazolidinyl urea
- DMDM hydantoin
- sodium hydroxymethylglycinate
- methenamine
- benzylhemiformal
- 5-bromo-5-nitro-1,3-dioxane

Isothiazolinone- and formaldehyde-free cosmetic brands include: Vanicream, Free & Clear, BaeBlu, Deciem, MooGoo, Nature's Gate, Derma E, Green People and Neal's Yard Remedies.

Isothiazolinone- and formaldehyde-free household brands include: Earthview, Eco-Me, Molly's Suds, Resparkle (Australia), Aspen Clean and Bio-D.

PPD allergy

One of the most dangerous allergens in cosmetics is para-phenylenediamine, or PPD, found in permanent hair dye blends.

Related chemicals, sometimes used in place of PPD in permanent hair dye products subsequently labeled PPD-free, include TD, TDS and PTD. Be aware that around half of people with PPD allergy also react to these alternatives.

There is a newer related chemical called ME+ (or ME-PPD) which is safer.

Nevertheless, you must be extremely careful with PPD allergies and take advice from your dermatologist.

Semi-permanent and temporary (generally henna-based) dyes may be your only options, although there are some more innovative approaches, including Hairprint.

Isothiazolinones are not commonly used in the hair dye blends themselves, but are sometimes included in the activators provided in hair dye kits, and also in the shampoo and/or conditioner sachets that can come with the package.

This is a large subject. There's a detailed article on the MI Free website which tells you more. Just search for 'PPD'.

Nickel / cobalt allergy

These common allergies, mostly affecting women, and often co-occurring, are largely due to prolonged exposure to metals and metal objects — through fastenings, coins, jewelry (especially piercings), watch straps / buckles, utensils, stationery, pins / needles, and in the case of cobalt, to dyes, inks, colors, ceramics / pottery, paints, and tools too.

They tend to be localized, only at the point of contact with the skin. You may be able to get some measure of protection by covering those points, either with band aids on the skin, or by using clear nail varnish (periodically applied) to the metal surface itself. However, avoidance is the safer solution. Avoid costume or cheap jewelry, and choose titanium covered razors, for instance.

In the EU, there are regulations restricting the degree to which nickel is permitted to leach from nickel-containing consumer products, and product recalls are issued for those which release too much.

There is no such regulation in the US, although this may change soon.

In cosmetics, cobalt compounds are used in some anti-perspirants and some hair dyes (typically light brown colors), so check ingredients for, usually, 'cobalt chloride'. Natural color rinses (eg henna) should be safe, as will many others.

Some foods happen to be high in nickel, although dietary sources only appear troublesome in those with particularly strong sensitivities. High-nickel foods include legumes / pulses (especially soya), black tea, coffee, chocolate, some nuts / seeds, wholegrains and canned food.

It's often advised to let water run through the tap before drinking from it.

Vitamin B12 contains cobalt, so you may react to a vitamin B12 injection.

Food hypersensitivities

These incorporate food allergy (which involves the immune system), celiac / coeliac disease (not a food allergy, strictly, but an autoimmune response to gluten), and food intolerances (which don't involve the immune system and cause digestive upsets, in the main).

These are managed by anything from strict avoidance in the case of the first two, and drastically reduced or moderated intake in the third.

If you are struggling to keep on top of your sensitivities, or find yourself reacting periodically, or are worried about your nutritional intake, then do consult your healthcare provider, and try to see a dietitian specialized in restricted diets.

Environmental allergies

Allergies to mold, pollen (hay fever), dust mite, and pet / animal dander can cause misery.

Use all the strategies at your disposal to help — air filters / purifiers, face masks, anti-histamines etc — many of which have been covered earlier in this book. Keeping on top of these will prevent over-challenging your immune system.

8. Emotional health

The psychological effects of eczema and skin allergies are not often discussed, and yet the impact on those with dermatitis and on their loved ones can be huge.

When so much of your life is spent on the practical realities of your condition — monitoring cosmetic labels, trying to keep away from exposures in unfamiliar places, applying topical medication — it's easy, but ultimately unwise, to neglect your or your child's emotional health.

Coping with diagnosis

Why me? Was it something I did wrong?

These are often your first thoughts upon confirmation of what you've perhaps suspected for a while. Be assured that in no way are you to blame for your allergy. You, or indeed your child, just got unlucky.

You may feel upset at this 'failure' of your body, and unable to take in the implications of what you've learned about MI allergy.

You may feel some relief at having answers, but in those who have been seeking a diagnosis for many months, that relief may be short-lived — the stress of not knowing what was wrong might now be replaced with the anxiety of managing the condition going forward.

It can be overwhelming.

Adopting a positive, can-do approach to the diagnosis can be helpful — and in buying this book, you clearly have the right attitude in looking to arm yourself with as much knowledge as you might need — but some, through no fault of their own, find the emotional road forward a tricky one.

Self-pity can be an initial issue, but a brief period spent feeling sorry for yourself can do you good. If you're overwhelmed with the diagnosis and its implications, having a short 'shut down' for a few days could be just what is needed, and is perfectly normal.

Anger and frustration are normal too. You may feel resentful of the situation in which you find yourself, and you may take your frustration out on loved ones. These feelings usually pass quickly.

Ongoing emotional problems

Some take skin allergies in their stride. Others experience occasional or chronic psychological problems or difficulties, and it is important to be aware of these possibilities.

Shame and stigma

Sadly, many feel embarrassed, even stigmatized, by their condition. Some report feeling like 'freaks' among acquaintances during flare-ups, when they may consider their condition unsightly and likely to attract unwelcome stares.

We live during a time when many are affected by low self-esteem, caused in part by the Instagram age of polished perfection. This impacts young people to a far greater degree.

Allergies — of all kinds — are not always understood well or taken seriously by members of the public, and this compounds the problem. People may be skeptical, unsympathetic, and may make you feel 'different'.

Those affected can react to this by avoiding social situations and isolating themselves, which is a cause for concern. Children can withdraw.

Depression

Symptoms of depression, some of which are applicable to children, include:

- indifference, including to pleasurable activities;
- lethargy and tiredness;
- disordered sleep and rest patterns;
- reduced appetite or, oppositely, comfort eating;
- low concentration and motivation;
- feelings of inadequacy, uselessness, hopelessness;
- loss of self-confidence;
- irritability and restlessness;
- withdrawal;
- lack of interaction with loved ones.

Anxiety and stress

These are common and often severe.

It's important to point out that some anxiety is important. From an evolutionary perspective, stress is a survivalist trait to keep you alert to possible danger and primed to respond to it. For instance, it is vital you maintain a low, constant level of vigilance to avoid exposure to your allergens. Don't look upon stress as all bad.

That said, chronic stress can be debilitating, and is a sign of a problem which needs resolving. Parents of allergic children can be extremely anxious — more so than they might be in their shoes. Stress also compounds asthma and eczema symptoms.

Symptoms of anxiety include:

- a dry mouth;
- cold or hot sweats;
- changes in eating habits;
- inability to work or concentrate;
- sleep disturbance;
- obviously untrue negative thoughts.

It can be a vicious circle: anxiety about your dermatitis or allergies can make the symptoms of it worse.

And worsening symptoms can worsen anxiety …

Self-help

So what to do?

Although there are plenty of individuals, specialists and groups who can help, you are undoubtedly the most important person involved in your own emotional care — or in that of your child.

Exercise

This does not necessarily mean going to the gym, or participating in sports you don't enjoy.

Run if you like, but walk if you don't. The key is movement through what makes you happy. Gardening, tennis, dance, even amateur dramatics, or playing with your dog — whatever gets you up and about.

There are too many benefits of exercise to itemize, not least for your heart and your emotional wellbeing, all of which have knock-on effects on other aspects of your health.

If you do strenuous exercise, and sweat a lot, be aware that this can aggravate some sensitive skins, as can the chemicals in swimming pools. Gentle but thorough cleansing, with all-important moisturization to follow, is always recommended.

Relaxation and breathing

Many claim they're unable to relax, but there is more to unwinding than merely willing yourself to do so.

Pampering — a warm bath, some candles — can help, as can a massage from a willing partner. Meditation, prayer and chanting are deeply relaxing; as are forms of yoga and healing martial arts such as t'ai chi. Find what works for you, and remember that relaxation takes practice.

For almost instant stress-relief if you're feeling anxious, try a technique of 'expanding' your peripheral vision:

- Find somewhere comfortable to sit, in relative quiet, where you won't be disturbed.

- Find a point opposite you, just above eye-level.

- Keeping your eyes fixed on that point, begin to slowly broaden your field of vision to notice more of what's on either side of the point.

- Keep going slowly until eventually you're paying attention to what is visible in the corners of your eyes.

- You should begin to feel your breathing moving lower in your chest, slowing down, becoming deeper, and your facial muscles relaxing.

This can be done for a few minutes several times a day, and will become more effective the more you do it.

Indeed, learning to breathe correctly is of great value to stress relief. Inhale deeply and slowly into the belly to the count of three, exhale evenly to the count of three, then pause for one — and repeat. Yogic breathing while seated and focussing on a lit candle is very soothing.

Sleep

Sleep is important for all-round health and wellbeing, but insomnia is a persistent issue for around one in four people. Here are some tips if you need them:

- Try to avoid eating too late, or too heavily, especially fatty meals, and go easy on alcohol and caffeine too.
- If your skin is hindering sleep, use emollient or any approach you've come to use for tackling itch and sensitivity.
- Stick to a regular sleep schedule: go to bed and get up at roughly the same time daily, in order to 'set' your body clock.
- Expose yourself to light during the day — perhaps combining it with some exercise — and ensure your home is well lit. Light exposure helps regulate sleep hormones.
- In the evening, avoid bright light from televisions, computers, e-readers, as well as domestic lighting.

- Also avoid too much stimulation — from your PC, television, or a thrilling book. Soft music or something soothing on the radio is better.

- A 'winding down' ritual can help: a warm bath or just getting changed into pyjamas and settling down with a warm drink can be enough — something you do in a relaxed atmosphere, perhaps by candlelight.

- Your bedroom should be cooler than your living room. If you ever sweat, it may be too warm; if you're tense in bed or find yourself hiding under the covers, it's too cool. Aim for around 16 degrees.

Knowledge

Learn everything you can about your allergies: your aim here is to eliminate the anxiety caused by the 'unknown'.

If there is something you do not understand, a niggling query which is bothering you, then resolve to find the answer. If this book can't help with it, ask a healthcare professional, or call an eczema charity, or post the question to a dedicated Facebook group. Whatever it takes.

Remind yourself that your allergy is, on the whole, manageable. You can develop avoidance strategies. You can treat symptoms when they occur. You will get better.

Try to actively learn from any reactions you have. Acknowledge that mistakes are human and natural. Forgive yourself for them. Accept that they may happen again, but that once again you will learn.

Positivity

Positive thinking helps your self-esteem and self-confidence, which may be dented by your allergic status. There will be situations when you will have to tell people about your allergy. Practice in front of a mirror if you are nervous about this. Or consider taking assertiveness classes if you feel this is a problem area. Never do it apologetically. You have nothing to be sorry for.

If you need evidence that attitudes are changing, take a look at the new 'skin positivity' movement which is picking up on social media, and which sets out to celebrate so-called imperfections in skin. It's an encouraging, emerging counter-trend to the glossy dominance of airbrushed flawlessness. It supports pride, acceptance, and encourages women (especially) to be more honest about their skin problems.

Volunteering

Helping yourself by helping others can work wonders.

Volunteering 'gives something back' to the allergy or skin community, and will also strengthen your character and prove deeply fulfilling.

If you have a dedicated skin or eczema charity in your country, perhaps contact its staff for suggestions and opportunities. For instance, the UK's National Eczema Society runs various support groups, and the US's National Eczema Association have an ambassador program where you can get involved with speaking, writing, events or social media.

You could perhaps consider other options, such as offering to give talks about skin allergies at your local school to children and teachers: it'll be rewarding to you, and informative for them.

Writing therapy

Putting your thoughts, anxieties and fears down on paper — be it print or virtual — is an excellent way of clearing your head, unburdening yourself, understanding your problems and charting your emotional progress.

Sharing your story of diagnosis or management with others can also help those newly diagnosed people currently going through the same thing.

You could start a blog — an online web diary of your experiences with allergy, which may well attract attention from other people worldwide who are in the same boat as you — or you could contribute a 'my story' to the MI Free website. (Write to me in the first instance at info@mi-free.com.)

Friends and family

The role of loved ones in your emotional care — or your own role in the care of your children — should never be underestimated.

Good friends ...

You need around you positive people who can offer practical advice and emotional support, who can bring light into your life when you feel there is none, and who make you feel understood.

The most valuable are those who know your needs, the implications of your allergy, can act as your personal 'bodyguards' should your guard slip — and who don't make any demands in return.

Shutting people out is a never-win situation. Most who care for you will want to help in any way they can, so don't be too proud to ask for practical help or a shoulder to cry on. You may feel you want to protect those close to you from the consequences or even burden of your allergy but, again, most prefer to be involved. Tell them what you need them to do for you. Do you think sticking to a particular air freshener in their home which you react to is *really* more important to them than your friendship and good health?

In the case of children, you may like to get their friends 'on side' too, perhaps working through their parents. Kids can relish the role of acting as supportive buddies to their friends — as is often the case with food allergies. They can help your child in situations where unfamiliar and potentially risky materials are introduced — for example, play slime, which may well be preserved with an isothiazolinone.

As a parent, you do of course have an important role — getting children to talk about their condition, right from the onset, at the point of diagnosis, by asking them how they feel. Start as you mean to go on. It will make dialogue easier in the future.

Family life can be deeply affected by allergy within the home. Non-allergic siblings can feel left out. Involve them if you can. Keeping isothiazolinone safe in the home is a team sport. You can get them interested in becoming label-aware, for example. Shared activities, doing things as a unit, can help solidify and forge closer ties between all. Don't neglect the simple basics of affection.

... and not so good friends

Understand that not everyone you meet, work with or are friendly with will be helpful or supportive, often through ignorance not malice.

Some people just don't *get* allergy, and will hold the view that 'allergies are all in the mind'. Upsetting as this may be, this will probably always be the way to some extent, and arguing the case may not always prove fruitful. The braver among you might like to show doubters pictures of your skin at its worst and most reactive state, but convincing them might not make you feel better.

All friends have their strengths and weaknesses, and a much valued confidante may not necessarily be the right one to turn to when you're suffering problems related to your allergy. Watch out for those who trivialize your allergy and tell you not to be silly, or who tell you about their problems with ill health when you ask for support with yours, or who appear bored by or indifferent towards your allergy.

Avoidance may be the best strategy when it comes to dealing with uncomprehending individuals such as work colleagues.

Children can be at risk of isolation at school if their allergies are severe. They may be teased or even bullied, especially if the school is visibly seen to be giving 'special treatment' to them. Their performance and mood may be effected. While it's important not to be too over-bearing or over-protective, it's worth keeping an eye on the situation, and talking gently to children about their friends, school life and social life. Get teachers involved if needs be.

Support groups

Occasionally, you may feel more comfortable seeking the support of strangers rather than that of loved ones.

Charities

Allergy charities generally have superb support lines manned by knowledgeable people who can offer emotional as well as practical guidance. See Resources on page 95.

Online support groups

A number of niche groups dedicated to people with allergy have sprung up online — including dedicated to MI.

People who live in secluded areas and feel isolated, those who are disabled, or single parents of young children, are among those who find these of particular value — but they can help anyone who is perhaps shy or has difficulty with face-to-face or voice-to-voice contact, and prefers the anonymity the web can offer.

Although groups can be encouraging and supportive, be sure to choose one with a knowledgeable moderator or administrator, who will remove any suspect, offensive or unsafe postings. Some have certain rules (for example, self-advertising or posting product recommendations may not be allowed) so acquaint yourselves with these before signing up or taking part.

Again, see Resources for links. Always try to 'give' as well as 'receive'. Ask for help, by all means, but also share advice and support others who ask for help at a later date.

Professional help

Sometimes, stubborn psychological problems need to be taken a step further.

Medical experts should be asking you about the psychological impact of your skin or your child's skin. Don't be afraid to broach the subject if no medical expert does. Ask who you can speak to about it.

We know from studies that supporting patients to find the right words to explain their symptoms and feelings can, for instance, help them become far more comfortable in their own skin, and less likely to feel self-conscious in public. If you're limiting your life because of your skin allergy, they are in an ideal position to help talk you through it.

Also, experts can help you come to terms with the fact that symptoms may re-occur, and that future reactions are possible.

If you're struggling to accept this, or you are worried about the severity of your next reaction, or you fear developing further allergies, let practitioners know.

Your doctor

Doctors might be your first port of call if you're experiencing symptoms of stress, depression, anxiety, or are concerned with other areas of your or your child's psychological health.

Doctors are trained to see signs of emotional difficulties in patients, and are ideally placed to advise on possible private treatments or referrals.

Many doctors have good counselling skills and unburdening yourself to one may be all you need.

Your dermatologist / allergy consultant

Your most complex queries can almost certainly be answered by your dermatologist or allergist, with whom you should try to develop a strong relationship.

The more knowledge you demonstrate, and the more questions you ask of specialists, the more likely you will be given greater detail and reassurance. If you feel burdened by not knowing whether or not you are newly allergic to a particular ingredient, for instance, a consultant can arrange further testing.

'Talking' therapists

If a doctor feels you need more specialized help, referral for counselling or psychotherapy may be suggested.

There are few differences between the talking therapies, even though counselling sounds — and is — gentler and less demanding than psychotherapy. Both involve face-to-face meetings with a trained therapist to reach any number of end goals, depending entirely on the patient, such as the reduction of psychological distress and the promotion of emotional health.

Counsellors will listen to you, aim to identify with you and your dilemmas, help you clarify them in your mind, and perhaps give advice — although generally their aim is to guide you to discover your own answers to your problems through carefully guided discussion. Counsellors can, for instance, help patients cope and come to terms with difficult events like diagnosis.

Psychotherapists, of which there are many kinds, work similarly, but use more analytical approaches and explore difficulties in greater depth. They may work with those with depression, anxiety and addictive behavior disorders, those who are finding it difficult to adjust to allergic illness, or those whose condition is impacting on many areas of their life.

Make sure you have an assessment session, and discontinue any therapy with a specialist with whom you feel uncomfortable — being at ease with your counsellor is vital. Remember too that counselling is not easy, nor a magic wand: expect positive changes but not miracles. Some people approach therapy expecting their stresses to be entirely removed, but therapists will not do this: they will arm you with coping mechanisms, not seek to abolish all your responses.

Accept recommendations from your medical practitioners, so that only suitably qualified individuals are recommended.

Cognitive Behavior Therapy (CBT)

CBT is an objective psychotherapeutic approach which is less interested in what caused your emotional difficulties, and more concerned with how you handle dilemmas.

It challenges the negative thought patterns which may be causing your problems, helps you identify and understand them, equips you with coping skills, and implements changes to unhelpful thinking or behavior. The therapy is structured, practical and result-focused, unlike counselling which usually involves 'freer' conversation and a greater rapport with the therapist.

CBT might be right for those looking for help with a specific issue. It is useful for depression, phobias or stress, for example, where the emphasis may be on cognition or thinking.

Hypnotherapy

This is a psychotherapy which uses hypnosis — a state of deep relaxation and heightened awareness, which makes the mind more receptive to positive suggestion. It can help those experiencing low self-esteem, anxiety and OCD, to name a few.

Conclusion: the outlook

Is the outlook for those with MI allergy a positive one — and what can those with MI allergy to do help?

Medical / research developments

Research into MI and related allergies is ongoing.

Some of it, perhaps frustratingly, has been centered on demonstrating the safety of isothiazolinones in certain circumstances, but a lot of studies have looked at, for instance, their cross-reactivity (their relationship to other allergens, and how likely people are to react to them if they react to isothiazolinones), and their environmental toxicity.

Cures, or even specific treatments, appear to be some way off, though. Although immunotherapy — desensitization therapy — has become available in some parts of the world for certain allergies (such as pollen), and has been looked at for some contact allergens, such as nickel, it hasn't really been successful and is not yet available.

Consumer tools

Newly diagnosed individuals, with many forms of atopic contact dermatitis, have few innovative tools at their disposal to help them stay healthy. More phone apps might help, and can be expected in future, but also analysis tools, such as chemical litmus-type or 'spot test' detection kits that already exist for allergens such as nickel, would be useful for those with allergy to isothiazolinones too.

Legislative improvements

The current research appears to be showing that it is through household detergents and products that sensitization to the isothiazolinones is increasingly occurring. This is possibly in part a consequence of the tightening of regulations on their use in cosmetics, especially in leave-on products.

More awareness is probably also driving cosmetic scientists to reformulate skincare products, and more clarity in labeling is helping reduce the risk too.

It is in household products that further improvements are required with regards to labeling and restrictions on permitted quantities of isothiazolinones, and there are signs that this may come soon.

Reporting reactions

If you have been sensitized by an isothiazolinone in a particular product, and this has been medically confirmed, it is worth contacting the manufacturer to let them know what has happened.

Do this in writing. Try to be calm and stick to known facts. By all means back up your letter with medical letters or reports and even photographs of your skin. It is important for brands to be aware when consumers react severely to their products and quality of life is deeply compromised.

However, if you were using several isothiazolinone-containing products prior to diagnosis, it may not be possible to confidently single out one as the cause. Playing the 'blame' game in this situation is arguably unfair, and remember that manufacturers are (almost always) operating within the laws.

You should also submit a report when you have a new reaction to an MI-free product you've been using. It could be a new allergy, or some other problem with the cosmetic or detergent, such as inappropriately high levels of a particular ingredient. Again, stick to the facts. Explain your situation, your *known* diagnosed allergens, and explain in detail what has happened.

You may think your one report may not achieve much, but if many other similar ones are received for the same product, brands will be alerted to a potential national or international problem.

Furthermore, brands may decide to look closely at their formulations, consult chemists or other experts, and perhaps reformulate products to the benefit of all consumers. This kind of reporting can also eventually generate a demand for more research investment in safer products.

In the UK / EU, it is obligatory for a brand's so-called Responsible Person to register any reported incident and transmit serious reports to relevant authorities. They are legally required to record and investigate undesirable effects.

Elsewhere, as well as writing to or calling the brands, it may well also be appropriate to report to authorities.

In the US, you can do this via the FDA's 'How to Report a Cosmetic Related Complaint' page on their website (www.fda.gov/cosmetics/complianceenforcement/adverseeventreporting/default.htm).

In Canada, you can report an incident involving a consumer product or cosmetic to Health Canada at www.canada.ca/en/health-canada/services/consumer-product-safety/advisories-warnings-recalls/report-incident-involving-consumer-product.html

The Allergy to Isothiazolinone, Methylisothiazolinone and Benzisothiazolinone Facebook group has a very helpful guide to reporting reactions to several authorities in a number of

countries. Find it at
www.facebook.com/notes/82101637795 2067/

Should isothiazolinones be banned?

It is understandable that many allergy advocates believe that isothiazolinones should be banned altogether, across all types of products, given the damage these preservatives have caused.

This is a contentious issue, however, and not as much of a no-brainer as it may appear.

The problem is that many industries are running out of preservatives, given some have already been banned, and others (such as parabens) have acquired an unjustified negative reputation. Abolishing isothiazolinones would result in an increased reliance on alternatives, risking more occurrence of sensitization to those, and further jeopardizing the health of others through new allergies.

We run the risk, long term, of having too few preservatives to turn to.

It is a debate which will probably run and run, at least until new preservatives are developed. They can't come too soon.

That said, urgently needed is the worldwide banning of MI and MCI in leave-on cosmetics. Where Europe has led, others must follow.

Also urgently needed without question is fully transparent and complete labeling — on all products, without exception.

After years of suffering, it's the absolute least which the isothiazolinone allergy community deserves.

Resources

Online groups

Methylisothiazolinone Free

This is the website and blog which I edit, and which inspired this book. You can find it at www.mi-free.com. It also has its own Facebook page (at www.facebook.com/mifree), and Twitter account (at www.twitter.com/freefrommi).

Allergy to Isothiazolinone, Methylisothiazolinone and Benzisothiazolinone

Excellent Facebook community, with large membership of around 10,000 worldwide, including a highly knowledgeable and supportive administrator, and albums of safe (and unsafe) products. Also includes useful articles on sunscreens and paints and regulatory news and more. It's an open group, but also offers a private group discussion which you can join. Find it at www.facebook.com/Allergy-to-Isothiazolinone-Methylisothiazolinone-and-Benzisothiazolinone-307128722674171

Methylisothiazolinone Victims

A public group described as 'a forum for discussion and support for anyone coping with an allergy or reaction to methylisothiazolinone'. Emphasis is less on products and more on product avoidance and minimalism, advocating a more natural, 'zero tolerance' approach to getting well. Again, knowledgeably administered, and boasting some useful information files, including on other allergies (eg Balsam of Peru, fragrance). Find it at www.facebook.com/groups/MIVictims

Methylisothiazolinone Allergy Support

A closed group "for those who have been patch tested and diagnosed with allergic contact dermatitis (ACD)/Type IV immune system delayed hypersensitivity to methylisothiazolinone or an other isothiazolinone". Find it at www.facebook.com/groups/217012078465804

Methylisothiazolinone Allergy Australia

"A group for sharing products with methylisothiazolinone and safer alternatives". Also a closed group. Find it at www.facebook.com/groups/MIAllergyAustralia

Charities

National Eczema Association (US)

A huge resource of advice and information. Can help you to find eczema experts. The NEA's mission is 'to improve the health and quality of life for individuals with eczema through research, support, and education'.

See: www.nationaleczema.org

Eczema Society of Canada

Dedicated to improving the lives of Canadians living with eczema. Advice on treatment, skincare products, finding a doctor and much more. Site has a list of organizations which can help with mental health issues.

See www.eczemahelp.ca

National Eczema Society (UK)

UK charity which focuses on giving advice on treatment and management — and on raising awareness.

See www.eczema.org

Eczema Association of Australasia

Dedicated to eczema patients in Australia, offering 'help, support, education and relief'.

See www.eczema.org.au

Professional organizations

American Contact Dermatitis Society

Mission: " … to promote, support, develop and stimulate information about contact dermatitis and occupational skin disease for improved patient care".

See www.contactderm.org

British Society for Cutaneous Allergy

British society which "promotes knowledge and best practice for the diagnosis and management of contact dermatitis".

See cutaneousallergy.org

European Society of Contact Dermatitis

Promotes "interest, stimulates research, and disseminates information on all aspects of contact dermatitis and other environmental and occupational skin diseases".

See www.escd.org

Miscellaneous

SkinSAFE

Cosmetic and household ingredient database, conceived in partnership with Mayo Clinic, enabling users to search safe products free from their triggers, including MI / MCI, among many others.

See www.skinsafeproducts.com

An app is also available.

See allergyfreeskin.com

Household Products Database

This is a US Department of Health & Human Services resource allowing you to search a) ingredients and find products containing them, and b) products you may be interested in, and the ingredients in them. It can be useful for tracking down suggestions for unusual types of products (browse the 'Types of Products' option), but it is not an exhaustive database, and complete ingredients are not always given. Use with caution, then, and as an additional tool, bearing in mind you may need to make further enquiries with manufacturers or stockists.

See hpd.nlm.nih.gov

Glossary

Names of isothiazolinones

Methylisothiazolinone and other isothiazolinone preservatives can appear in a number of guises.

Common names
Here is a non-exhaustive list:

- Methylisothiazolinone (MI / MIT)
- Methylchloroisothiazolinone (MCI / MCIT)

- Benzisothiazolinone (BIT)
- Chloromethylisothiazolinone (CMIT) (alternative name for methylchloroisothiazolinone)
- Octylisothiazolinone (OIT, OI)

- Butyl-benzisothiazolinone (BBIT)
- Dichloro-octylisothiazolinone (DCOIT)
- Dichloro-methylisothiazolinone (DCMIT)

The first two above are the most common expressions you'll encounter for the two main isothiazolinone preservatives. Only these two names will be seen on cosmetics in the EU, and generally in North America and Australia too — although sometimes you may also see Kathon CG (Kathon Cosmetic

Grade — listed below). They may also appear on other products, such as household detergents.

These two are most commonly seen on household products, along with the subsequent second group of three names above.

The final group of three are rare, newer isothiazolinone preservatives, which may become more common in future, albeit not in cosmetics.

Chemical names

These include:

- 1,2-benzisothiazol-3(2H)-one
- 2-methyl-4-isothiazol
- 2-methyl-4-isothiazolin-3-one
- 5-chloro-2-methyl-4-isothiazolin-3-one
- chloro-2-methyl-3-(2H)-isothiazolinone

… and many similar variations.

These are rarely seen on products, but may appear in, for example, material safety data sheets (MSDSs), such as those produced for paints.

It's important if you check with producers of non-cosmetic products that they understand that the isothiazolinone preservatives can appear under these and other variations.

If you need to scrutinize lists of ingredients, check for the "isothiazol" string of letters, which is the usual tell-tale sign, among all the numbers, brackets and hyphens.

That said, some paint manufacturers refer to the preservatives as "thiazoles" or "thiazoline compounds", so watch out for these too.

Brand names

There are many branded preservative mixes which include one or more of the isothiazolinone preservatives.

Again, these may be seen on MSDSs, and again they pose a danger because unwitting customer service agents may not be aware of what exactly they represent. If you can, ask for the full preservation system used in the product — and look it up if necessary.

This list below is by no means exhaustive and new ones regularly come onto the market.

In some cases, there are often many letter / number combinations following the name, denoting additional varieties, so only one or two examples of each are given.

- Acticide MBS / MBR
- Algucid CH50
- Amerstat 250
- Euxyl K 100
- Fennosan IT 21
- Grotan K / TK2
- IPX
- Isocil® PC
- Kathon CG / LX / WT
- Koralone B-119 / B-120 / N-105
- Mergal K7
- Metatin GT
- Mitco CC 31/32 L
- Neolone CapG / 950 / MxP

- Nipacide CFX
- Parmetol A / DF / K
- Piror P109
- Promex Alpha / BM
- Proxan
- Proxel AQ / CRL / PL / XL2
- Skane M-8
- Special Mx 323

CAS (Chemical Abstracts Service) numbers

These may appear on Material Safety Data Sheets instead of a name:

- 2682-20-4 — Methylisothiazolinone (MI)
- 26172-55-4 — Methylchloroisothiazolinone (MCI)
- 55965-84-9 — MI / MCI blend (ie Kathon CG)
- 2634-33-5 — Benzisothiazolinone (BIT)
- 26530-20-1 — Octylisothiazolinone (OIT)

These and other CAS numbers for more obscure isothiazolinone preservatives can be viewed at www.chemicalland21.com/lifescience/phar/5-CHLORO-2-METHYL-3(2H)-ISOTHIAZOLONE.htm

Safe ingredients

As outlined in the book, there is always the possibility that if you react to one or more of the isothiazolinones, you may react to other ingredients, such as other preservatives, or fragrances in cosmetics and household goods.

However, the following non-isothiazolinone preservatives, should be safe for you:

- Benzyl alcohol
- Diazolidinyl urea
- Ethylhexylglycerin
- Imadozolidinyl urea
- Levulinic acid
- Parabens (such as methylparaben, propylparaben)
- Phenoxyethanol
- Potassium sorbate / sorbic acid
- Sodium benzoate / benzoic acid
- Sodium salicylate
- Tetrasodium EDTA
- Triclosan

And many others …

False enemies

You may also encounter some ingredients whose names may resemble methylisothiazolinone — or other isothiazolinones — but are in fact fine.

These 'false enemies' include:

- Methyl benzoate

- Methyleugenol
- Methylpropanediol
- Methylpropional
- Methyl sulfonyl methane
- Methylparaben

Again, you need to concern yourself with the giveaway "isothiazol" string of letters, *not* necessarily the "methyl".

The fragrance compound alpha isomethyl ionone (or just 'isomethylionone') is also *not* related to the isothiazolinones, and should be safe.

Acknowledgements

Thanks have to go to the isothiazolinone allergy community online, from whom I've learned much of what I know. Many of their tips and experiences have fed this book, and I couldn't have written much of it without them.

Thanks too to those who have subscribed to my website, who have interacted with me, and who have sent me useful links and info. There are too many to name, and if I try I will omit some who don't deserve it, but I appreciate all.

I'd like to express huge gratitude to Dana Todd, who read most of the key chapters and gave me invaluable feedback. *Living with Methylisothiazolinone Allergy* would have been a much poorer book without her highly knowledgeable input, and I'm extremely grateful for her work on it.

Thanks too to Michelle, who gave me the nudge I needed to finish *LwMA*, just when I was beginning to wonder whether I ever would.

Cover image credit: congerdesign / Pixabay (congerdesign@web.de)

Index

air conditioning 45, 51

air fresheners 45

air purifiers / filters 44–5

allergic contact dermatitis (ACD) 3

allergy 2–3; *see also* food allergy, environmental allergy *and* isothiazolinones, allergy to

American Contact Dermatitis Society xiii, 97

anaphylaxis 5

antibiotics 49, 57

anti-histamines 55–6

anxiety 77–8

asthma 5

barrier methods 39–45

bathing 59–62

benzisothiazolinone ix, 1, 18, 29; *see also* isothiazolinones

bleach baths 59–61

breathing 79–80 *see also* asthma *and* masks, facial

charities 85, 95–6

children 47, 84–5

cleaning agents *see* cosmetics *and/or* household products

clothing, exposure through 52
clothing, protective 42–3 *see also* gloves
cobalt, allergy to 73–4
cognitive behavior therapy 88–9
contact dermatitis 3; systemic 5
cortisone / corticosteroids 15, 56, 57
Cosmetic Ingredient Review x
cosmetics 17; as barriers 39–40; as treatments 58; fragrance free 25, 70; hypoallergenic 22–3, 25; ingredients on 17; isothiazolinone-free 24–5; labelling of 17–20; regulations ix–xii, xiv, 18–19, 26, 27–8, 91
Cosmetics Europe xiv
counselling 87–8

depression 77
dermatitis, contact *see* contact dermatitis
dermatologist 87
detergents, household *see* household products
diagnosis, of isothiazolinone allergy 7–15; coping with 75–6
diet 64–5
doctor 8–9, 87

emotional health 75–89
environmental allergy 74
essential oils 21, 68, 69
European Commission xiii–xiv

exercise 78–9

exposure to isothiazolinones; avoidance of 39–54; in cosmetics ix–xiv, 1, 2; in household products 1, 2; in public places 45–52; occupational ix, 10, 46

Food & Drug Administration (FDA) 18, 22, 93

food allergy 3, 74

formaldehyde; allergy to 70–2; cosmetics free from 72; household products free from 72

fragrance 20–2; allergy to 67–9; ingredients in 20–1; isothiazolinones in 20–1

fragrance allergens 23, 69, allergy to 68–9; in cosmetics 20–3; in household products 30

fragrance free 20, 67, 70

'free from' claims 18

friends and family 83–5

furniture 53

gloves 40–2

goggles 44

hair treatments 51–2, 72; *see also* cosmetics

history, of isothiazolinones ix–xiv

holidays 50–1

hospital treatment 48–9

household products 29–38; fragrance free 70; homemade 34–6; hypoallergenic 33; isothiazolinone free 30, 33–4; isothiazolinones used in 1, labeling of 30–2

hypnotherapy 89

hypoallergenic *see* cosmetics, hypoallergenic *and/or* household products, hypoallergenic

immuno-modulators 56

immuno-suppressants 15, 57

isothiazolinones ix, 1; allergy symptoms caused by 4–5, 62–3; allergy to 2–3; alternative names for 99–102; effectiveness of 2; permitted concentrations of x, xii, xiv, 27–8; use of ix–xiv, 1–2; *see also* benzisothiazolinone, methylchloroisothiazolinone, methylisothiazolinone *and/or* octylisothiazolinone

Kathon CG (MI / MCI blend) ix–x, xii, xiv, 1, 2, 18, 28, 99–100; *see also* isothiazolinones

labeling, cosmetics *see* cosmetics, labeling of

labeling, household products *see* household products, labeling of

laundry products *see* household products

legislation, cosmetics *see* cosmetics regulations

masks, facial 43

material safety data sheets (MSDS) 10, 32, 100

medical treatment 48–9

medication 55–7

menopause 4

methylchloroisothiazolinone ix, xii, 1; allergy to ix, 2; *see also* Kathon CG *and* isothiazolinones

methyldibromo glutaronitrile (MDBGN) x–xi

methylisothiazolinone ix, xii–xiii, 1; allergy to ix, 2; *see also* isothiazolinones

nickel, allergy to 73, 91

octylisothiazolinone ix, 1, 29; *see also* isothiazolinones

paint(s) 1, 29, 36–7, 43, 45; neutralising wash for 37–8

parabens xi, 2

parfum 20–2, 69 *see also* fragrance *and* fragrance allergens

patch testing 9–14; contra-indications 9–10; of fragrance 68–9; side effects 13, 14

phototherapy 57

PPD, allergy to 72

preservatives 94, 102–3 *see also* formaldehyde, isothiazolinones *and/or* parabens

prevalence, of allergy to isothiazolinones 3

printers / printer ink 46

psychotherapy 88–9

public transport 48

reactions; reporting of 92–4; to isothiazolinones *see* symptoms of isothiazolinone allergy

regulations, cosmetic *see* cosmetics regulations

relaxation 79–80

safety data sheets *see* material safety data sheets

school 47, 85

self-diagnosis 7–8

sensitization (allergic) 3

skin allergy *see* contact dermatitis

sleep 80–1

soap 19, 58

societies, professional / dermatological 97–8

steroids *see* corticosteroids

stress 77–8

support groups 85–6, 95–7

symptoms, of isothiazolinone allergy 4–5; monitoring of 8–9; return of 62–3

talking therapy 87–9

tattoos 52

tests, for allergy *see* patch testing

travel 27

treatment, for isothiazolinone allergy 55-64, 91

type I allergy 3

type IV allergy 3, 55

volatile organic compounds (VOCs) 37, 43
volunteering 82

writing therapy 82–3